THE GROWTH

OF MEDICAL THOUGHT

The Growth

of Medical Thought

LESTER S. KING, M.D.

THE UNIVERSITY OF CHICAGO PRESS

The University of Chicago Press, Chicago 60637
The University of Chicago Press, Ltd., London

International Standard Book Number: 0-226-43703-5
Library of Congress Catalog Card Number: 63-9729

*To scholars, whose achievements
we appreciate only when we try to follow
in their footsteps*

Preface

Medical history has no definable limits. When we regard the medical scene, we find reflected there innumerable facets of human knowledge. Many different elements—cultural and philosophic, political, scientific, socio-economic—have left their traces upon medicine, so that a truly comprehensive medical history would need be a history of civilization. It is obvious that no one can write such a history. At best we can describe only a limited area, from a limited point of view.

My own interests center not so much on the great medical achievements as on the concepts and ideas that have influenced medicine. I have found especially fascinating the ways in which doctors have tried to explain disease. The explanations which one era accepted readily seem grossly inadequate to another era, because the ideas and attitudes and the whole intellectual climate have changed. The history of medicine is part of the history of ideas. The medical world is indeed a microcosm which reproduces *in parvo* a vast macrocosm of concepts and thoughts.

At irregular intervals great discoveries have changed the whole course of medicine, but the intervening periods have not been static. They manifest a gestation of new ideas and a struggle between new concepts and the old established doctrines. I have tried to study problems sympathetically, to indicate the difficulties involved, and render them meaningful to present-day interests. From the great men who have studied the causes of disease I have selected a few representatives and tried to present their thinking in a manner relevant to their own setting yet consonant with present-day idiom.

I offer no apologies for the particular selection of authors and of eras. Other historians would doubtless have chosen quite differently, but my own choice offers what seems an appropriate framework for a broad survey. Each chapter discusses a separate historical period, and each of them would demand a lifetime for adequate mastery. Quite obviously I have made no effort at exhaustive coverage; if scholars choose to point out relevant material which I have neglected, I must plead guilty in advance. But my purpose was not to give a complete history. Choosing a few individuals who represent trends in intellectual history, I have tried by episodic treatment to indicate the growth of medical science and the patterns of medical doctrine. I have tried to place in perspective the critical spirit and sound method that good physicians have displayed throughout history, and also to show the pitfalls that beset even the wisest.

How to explain disease is a task as important today as it was 2,500 years ago. In attempting to solve the persistent problems of disease, investigators have been forced to rephrase their questions. And as the questions have assumed different forms, so too have the answers. In order to understand today's answers we must understand yesterday's questions, and the answers given then.

It is a pleasure to acknowledge the help which I have received from so many sources. I particularly want to thank Dr. Walter Pagel who, in correspondence and in personal discussion, shared with me his profound and unmatched knowledge of Paracelsus. However, for all interpretations appearing in this book the responsibility is exclusively mine. I want also to thank the library staffs at the University of Illinois, The John Crerar Library, the University of Chicago, and Northwestern University, who made my task so much easier. My secretary, Mrs. Cynthia Azar, has shown uncanny ability in reading my handwriting and has cheerfully worked with me in the many revisions of the text. I want to acknowledge the courtesy of Blackwell Scientific Publications for permission to quote from Harvey's *The Circulation of the Blood* and *Movement of the Heart and Blood in Animals,* so excellently translated by Dr. Kenneth J. Franklin. And finally, I want to acknowledge gratefully the aid received from the U.S. Public Health Service. Part of the work which this book involved was supported by their research grant, R. G. 9214.

L. S. K.

Contents

Prologue

It is surprising, perhaps, to realize how many people at one time or another exert some sort of medical function. The old-world grandmother who nursed a dozen cases of measles in her own children does not hesitate to make a diagnosis on her young grandchild, nor to tell her daughter precisely what to do. The arthritic may sing the praises of flannel cloths and goose-fat; the newspaper editor may freely recommend a "reducing diet," and the pharmacist a sleeping-pill or headache remedy. Laymen who give such advice are relying on experience. Often the advice seems to work, perhaps not perfectly, but at least to a gratifying degree.

Many laymen have been extremely skilled in diagnosis and have achieved considerable therapeutic success. However, giving appropriate advice is only part of medical skill—an important practical part, to be sure, but still only a part. The layman can learn from experience what to do, but the physician must also know *why* he does what he does. He must know it in a manner quite detailed, clear and rational, organized and logical. It is this knowledge which sets off the physician from the layman. As we shall see, Aristotle made the distinction quite explicit, that almost anyone can learn procedure empirically, through rule of thumb, but whoever lays claim to scientific knowledge must know the reasons and the general principles.

There is a tremendous body of scientific knowledge which is the heritage of today's physician. As a student he begins to acquire a well-organized background which provides reasons for what he does, and his teachers hope that he will remain a student all his life. To a great degree medical knowledge centers on the problem, How do diseases arise? If we know how they come to be; if, in medical jargon, we know their "pathogenesis," our treatment will be "scientific," and not merely lucky. But we cannot understand pathogenesis unless we understand what factors are relevant to any given disease condition, and how these factors may operate.

Needless to say, our views of pathogenesis have changed over the centuries, as our knowledge of the world has changed. For example, the doctor today may look at that painful affliction called a boil, and try to explain it. He will talk about bacteria, and how they get into the tissues, and what they do when they get there. He will talk about staphylococcus aureus, inflammation, and pus, and the reactions of host and bacterium, and the phenomena of immunity and resistance. If he goes far enough into the minutiae of knowledge, he eventually may get lost in a jungle of biochemical reactions. But even if he does not wander so far, and is content to leave ultimate details to the specialist, he nevertheless knows the major principles, and is *rational*.

The historian points out that the current doctrine about boils is only one of many possible accounts. It is one particular explanation which became dominant only after bacteria were discovered. Yet long before staphylococci were discovered, men suffered from boils and sought some kind of explanation. Why do boils arise, and how? The Book of Job relates a well-known case history in considerable detail, with a scheme of pathogenesis. Succeeding eras have presented widely different sets of reasons, that is, different schemata of pathogenesis. The historian wants to know: What did doctors say before staphylococci were recognized? How did they explain a boil? What reasons did they give if their treatment was successful—or unsuccessful?

The doctor, then, is concerned with the problem, How do diseases arise? The historian faces a different problem, namely, At different times in history, how did people *say* that diseases arose? This is quite a different matter. Explanations have changed radically through the ages. Different cultural groups at different eras of history have offered quite different reasons for what they did. In any given disease the explanation which past generations offered may seem to us bizarre. While it is sometimes tempting, when describing the past, to emphasize the seeming absurdities, we must realize that the older physicians, when they brought forward their explanations, did so in good faith and with considerable confidence. If their explanations seem silly to us, we merely show our lack of historical appreciation. We must assume that ancient physicians were just as intelligent as we today, and that whatever they said and did, they said and did for good reasons. If we assume this, then the historical problem becomes: *What were those reasons* which they considered good?

How does it happen that they said one thing while we say another?

The explanations that we give have deep roots. Our answers derive from our entire way of life, our intellectual background, cultural heritage, and sense of values, so that an explanation may be a mirror which reflects the entire cultural setting. Problems have always evoked questions, and questions sooner or later produce answers which always flow from the contemporary beliefs. As Willey indicated,[1] an explanation may be considered a restatement of current interests or assumptions. This book is an attempt to study some of the presuppositions that entered into the medical background of times gone by, how these presuppositions led to particular explanations, and how explanations changed and led to modern medical science.

From Religion to Science

APOLLO, ASCLEPIUS, HIPPOCRATES

Life and death are such an important part of religion that the problems of disease readily find explanation within a religious framework. Religions, of course, have varied greatly. Those forces which one culture might call "natural," another might represent as the will of superhuman beings, of gods and goddesses who have human emotions and whose behavior patterns quite closely parallel human examples. It is a very human tendency to distribute rewards to express pleasure and punishments to express displeasure. If gods controlled the natural forces, they might be assumed to behave similarly. If pleased, the gods might send prosperity; if displeased, affliction. In such a formulation illness could represent a punishment reflecting the displeasure of a particular god against a particular person.

Greek mythology offers many examples of this theme, and the *Iliad* is indeed built around it. The Trojan War took place probably in the twelfth century B.C., while the *Iliad,* after a long oral tradition, was probably written down in the eighth century B.C. It thus reflects the culture of a considerable time span, and the corresponding attitudes toward disease.

As the poem opens, the Greeks had already besieged Troy for nine years. Agamemnon previously, at the sack of Thebes, had seized as captive the beautiful daughter of Chryses, the priest of Apollo. When Chryses with rich gifts tried to secure his daughter's freedom, Agamemnon not only refused to give her up, but roughly and disrespectfully sent the old priest away.

Then went that aged man apart and prayed aloud to kind Apollo. . . . "If ever I burnt to thee fat flesh of thighs of bulls or goats, fulfil thou this my desire; let the Danaäns pay by thine arrows for my tears."

So spake he in prayer, and Phoebus Apollo heard him and came down from the peaks of Olympus wroth at heart, bearing on his shoulders his bow and covered quiver. And the arrows clanged upon his shoulders in his wrath. . . . Then he . . . let an arrow fly; and there was heard a dread clanging of the silver bow. First did he assail the mules and fleet dogs, but afterward, aiming at the men his piercing dart, he smote; and the pyres of the dead burnt continually in multitudes.[1]

For nine days Apollo wrought destruction, and by the tenth day of the pestilence Achilles, inspired by Hera, tried to do something about it. The Greeks sought counsel of their own priests. One soothsayer declared that Apollo was angry because of Agamemnon's behavior toward Chryses. And *therefore*—it is important to note the causal connections—therefore Apollo "brought woes upon us, and will bring. Nor will he ever remove the loathly pestilence from the Danaäns till we have given the bright-eyed damsel to her father . . . and carried a holy hecatomb to Chryses; then might we propitiate him to our prayer."

This blunt diagnosis and the appropriate recommended therapy made Agamemnon very angry, for he did not want to give up the girl. But he finally agreed to do so, on condition that he receive in recompense the girl who was Achilles' prize. The idea infuriated Achilles, and strong words passed between the two warriors. Achilles had to submit, and the story of the *Iliad* concerns the outcome of this quarrel between Achilles and Agamemnon, a quarrel which involved the gods as well as the Greeks and the Trojans. For our purposes the later happenings are not relevant. The significant feature is that the soothsayer's advice was followed. The captive Chryseis was returned to her father, along with appropriate sacrifices to Apollo. After proper ceremonies the satisfied Chryses prayed again to Apollo, who then removed the pestilence.

Here then we have a complete epidemiological study, narrated in great detail. Clearly indicated are the causes, the mechanism, the diagnosis, and the remedy. How are we to regard it? One aspect that has interested modern scholars is, What *was* this plague that attacked the Greek host? How can the data of Homer be transposed into modern categories, so that present-day information can "explain" the facts which Homer set forth? In other words, if a modern doctor, with his present-day knowledge and concepts, had been at Troy, what would his diagnosis have been? Daremberg[2] in 1865 indicated that there were too few details to allow us to characterize the disease, and a century later this pronouncement still stands. But the very question, "What do *we* think of that disease?" is entirely foreign to the spirit of this book. The important question is, "What did *they* think of it?" We

7

want to find out how *their* minds worked, what elements of scientific method they exhibited, what their views of disease have in common with our own.

If we examine the narrative critically, we can appreciate two quite different types of assertions. One category we can loosely call "facts." While we do not know that they actually occurred, they very easily might have, and they are not in any way inconsistent with what we accept and believe today. Among these "facts" are: Agamemnon and Achilles had each captured very desirable maidens. Chryses, the father of Agamemnon's captive, sought his daughter's release. He was rebuffed. Chryses was a priest of Apollo. Chryses prayed to Apollo. A pestilence afflicted the Greek host, attacking first the animals and then the men. The Greeks restored the ravished daughter to Chryses. Chryses prayed again to Apollo. The pestilence ceased. All of these we may construe as "facts of observation" or data of experience. They represent a description about which there need be no dispute.

But other assertions are not so clear-cut. Homer said quite a lot about Apollo, what he did and how he reacted. These statements are rather distinct from those describing what Agamemnon did, and represent quite a different category. Actually, the Greeks did not see Apollo, or touch him, yet the god was considered to be quite real. It is, of course, quite logical to believe firmly that what we do not see is real, provided we have good grounds for doing so. When, for example, we press the light switch, we do not see the electric current. But we do see its effects, which are sufficiently impressive to induce complete belief in the reality of electricity. In the same way the Greeks accepted the reality of Apollo, not through bodily presence but through attributed effects.

We readily distinguish facts of direct observation from concepts which are inferred. The latter represent interpretation rather than direct observations. Thus, when we press the switch, the incandescent bulb is a directly observed fact, but the electric current is an inference, conceptual entity, or interpretation. In the same way, we think of Agamemnon as something directly observable, while Apollo is an inference or a concept.

Now Homer, while discussing the epidemic, used the concept "Apollo" to explain, or tie together, various of the observed data. It was because of Apollo that certain observed facts became intelligible, took on particular meaning, and exhibited a clear orderly relationship. It was Apollo who heard Chryses' prayer, became angry at the affront offered the priest, and responded by killing large numbers of Greeks. It was Apollo, again, who stopped the pestilence when the appeased Chryses so requested. In this epidemiological study, therefore, Apollo represents the explanatory concept. Hence, the properties or characteristics of Apollo are very relevant to understanding the epidemic.

Since in later chapters we will meet quite different types of explanation, it is worth while to note briefly and in rudimentary fashion what we mean by the explanatory process. For a truly rigorous analysis, the reader must plunge deeply into philosophy, for example, the superb recent volume of Nagel.[3]

At any given moment, or during any given time span, the number of facts, either observed or capable of observation, is virtually infinite. This is apparent when we try to diagnose an illness. For any patient, with any disease, the number of available "facts" is without limit—all the details of his past history from earliest infancy, including not only strictly medical factors, but his social and educational background, habits, occupation, and emotional experiences, may be significant. It may be extremely important to learn a great deal about his parents and siblings, as well as more remote relatives. A detailed physical examination can disclose innumerable bits of information. And what is not apparent to the unaided senses may be revealed by special examinations, the so-called "tests." And then, no matter how large the total mass of facts, it can always be increased.

Obviously in any given illness only relatively few data are significant. Some facts may seem to form a pattern, to exhibit a special relationship or inner connection which they share with each other, to which other data are irrelevant. Thus, in studying a patient, the physician may attend closely to the history of frequent sore throats, the presence of fever, joint pains and swelling, change in the quality and rhythm of the heart sounds. But the physician who notes these would disregard a mole on the chin, a history of measles at the age of three, a dislike of spinach, and the death of a grandfather in a train accident. The latter are equally facts but they do not fit into a perceived pattern. They are irrelevant.

The physician not only selects facts, but he fits them together into a pattern. By analogy, beads strung together are quite different from a loose miscellaneous heap, for the cord or thread has imposed a pattern or relationship which is maintained. In similar fashion the physician imposes order on his selected data by using an explanatory concept, in this case "rheumatic fever." This is the explanatory principle which renders the isolated data meaningful.

Let us return now to the *Iliad,* and study Homer's explanation. Homer, as an artist, had already discarded most of the irrelevant details. In telling his story he selected only those facts which were relevant, that is, which in his mind already exhibited an inner connection. He presented his story with the correlations already indicated. To tie the data together he utilized the concept of the god Apollo, a concept that was rich and meaningful.

However, while to the Greeks Apollo was real, to us he is only a myth. As scientists we cannot use myths to explain real events. We cannot string beads on an imaginary thread. When we look critically at the Homeric narrative, we can accept Agamemnon or the stricken soldiers as real. We can accept Chryses the priest, and can also accept the concept of gods. If *we* face the bare facts of the Homeric narrative, and try to explain them, we cannot place all the beads on a single thread.

To explain the Homeric narrative in modern terms, we would make a sharp discrimination. We would separate the data of illness—the dead soldiers and dogs and mules —from the prayers, rituals, and sacrifices. The actual disease we would try to make orderly by a concept "infectious agent, type unknown, perhaps a virus." Such a concept, however vague, nevertheless harmonizes with our twentieth-century intellectual background. On the other hand we would explain the various data of Homeric mythology through the terms of comparative religion, psychology, and anthropology. Whereas Homer saw a unified drama, with all parts intimately related in a single pattern, the modern temper finds two separate and disconnected series and two distinct explanatory concepts. The anger of a mythological being, however useful to explain disease three thousand years ago, is not accepted today.

II

Apollo served Greek medicine not merely as a god who might send disease or cure it but also as the father of Asclepius, the god of healing. In this regard, historians owe a profound debt to the Edelsteins, whose work on Asclepius is now the definitive source-book.[4]

There are many myths about the life of Asclepius. They differ one from the other but all have a central theme: Coronis was the mother of Asclepius and Apollo his father; Coronis was not faithful to Apollo, and the god therefore brought about her death. According to Ovid, Apollo himself transfixed her with one of his arrows, but whether he himself executed the punishment, or merely decreed her death, is not so important. The accounts agree that when Coronis was on her funeral pyre Apollo rescued the unborn babe and entrusted him to Chiron the Centaur, who taught him the arts of medicine. Asclepius became a great physician, but was finally killed by Jove's thunderbolt for bringing a dead man back to life. Whether he did this for gain, with venal motives, or did it as the highest achievement of medical art, is a moot point.

Asclepius as a person is a very shadowy figure. Apart from his medical skill his personality is rather a blank. Other mythological figures have a decided personality, and rather precise characterization, but Asclepius serves merely to express an idea: "All his being is integrated into one function, that of healing and helping mankind."[5]

In earlier literature Asclepius was a mortal, a hero but not a god, but he became transformed into the god of medicine, preserver of health, and an object of reverence and worship. To him prayers might be offered, hymns sung, festivals celebrated. There were temples devoted to the god, the most important of which were at Epidaurus, Cos, and Pergamos. The visitor to Greece today may see the ruins, partly restored, where the treatments took place.

It seems generally agreed that the patients who sought the god's help in the temples first had to bathe, and also offer sacrifices, which might be quite humble. Special fasts or rites of purification were not necessary. Most important, however, was the "temple sleep" and the accompanying dreams which the patients experienced in the *abaton,* or sleeping-room. Of the many records describing these experiences, most famous are the inscriptions found at Epidaurus. It is worth while to quote entire certain of these, thought to date from the second half of the fourth century B.C.:

8. Euphanes, a boy of Epidaurus. Suffering from stone he slept in the temple. It seemed to him that the god stood by him and asked: "What will you give me if I cure you?" "Ten dice," he answered. The god laughed and said to him that he could cure him. When day came he walked out sound.

18. Alcetas of Halieis. This blind man saw a dream. It seemed to him that the god came up to him and with his fingers opened his eyes, and that he first saw the trees in the sanctuary. At daybreak he walked out sound.

28. Cleinatas of Thebes with the lice. He came with a great number of lice on his body, slept in the Temple, and sees a vision. It seems to him that the god stript him and made him stand upright, naked, and with a broom brushed the lice from off his body. When day came he left the Temple well.

36. Cephisias . . . with the foot. He laughed at the cures of Asclepius and said: "If the god says he has healed lame people he is lying; for, if he had the power to do so, why has he not healed Hephaestus?" But the god did not conceal that he was inflicting penalty for the insolence. For Cephisias, when riding, was stricken by a bullheaded horse which had been tickled in the seat, so that instantly his foot was crippled and on a stretcher he was carried into the Temple. Later on, after he had entreated him earnestly, the god made him well.[6]

The significant feature in this type of inscription is, that the god personally brought about a cure in the suppliant patient. Preliminary conditions had to be met, yet the essence of the cure is *the personal relationship between the god and the particular patient*. The will of the god acts directly on a single individual.

In other inscriptions there was a changed relationship.

For example, in the second century A.D. we encounter the following case records:

To Lucius who suffered from pleurisy and had been despaired of by all men the god revealed that he should go and from the threefold altar lift ashes and mix them thoroughly with wine and lay them on his side. And he was saved and publicly offered thanks to the god, and the people rejoiced with him.

To Julian who was spitting up blood and had been despaired of by all men the god revealed that he should go and from the threefold altar take the seeds of a pine cone and eat them with honey for three days. And he was saved and went and publicly offered thanks before the people.

To Valerius Aper, a blind soldier, the god revealed that he should go and take the blood of a white cock along with honey and compound an eye salve and for three days should apply it to his eyes. And he could see again and went and publicly offered thanks to the god.[7]

These latter testimonies show the god acting as a physician, that is, one who prescribed a drug effective in curing the particular disease. Cure was not merely through divine fiat. The cure was wrought by medicine, while the god indicated which medicine was appropriate to the particular condition. The treatment was still highly personalized, for there was no implication that the next patient who entered the temple with a similar complaint would receive the same advice. There was no declaration that every case of hemoptysis should be treated by honey and pine cones, no universal formulation that all cases of a given type should receive a specified treatment. But there was the significant feature that the actual cure was wrought by medicine.

Inscriptions such as these suggest a transition to natural science. When a god acts by fiat, it is his will that brings about the desired result. When Apollo willed a pestilence to afflict the Greeks, his arrows instrumented his will. Yet arrows per se do not carry pestilence. They do so only when the god so wills it. When the god brushed away the lice to produce a cure, it was the god's will which produced the cure, not the mechanical act of brushing. The concept of a medicine, however, indicates some sort of a curative power inherent in the object. It is the drug which cures, but the god indicates what drug should be used. The god no longer has such complete power that he can accomplish his aims merely by fiat.

This is indicated in the following testimony (first century B.C.):

> When for two years I had coughed incessantly so that I discharged purulent and bloody pieces of flesh all day long, the god took in hand to cure me. . . . He gave me rocket to nibble on an empty stomach, then Italian wine flavored with pepper to drink, then again starch with hot water, then powder of the holy ashes and some holy water, then an egg and pine-resin, then again moist pitch, then iris with honey, then a quince and a wild purslane to be boiled together—the fluid to be drunk, while the quince was to be eaten—then to eat a fig with holy ashes taken from the altar where they sacrificed to the god.[8]

Surely a roundabout method of producing a cure. If the god could heal merely by an act of will, why make the procedure so complicated? But in this case it seems that the god must work through natural objects.

A religious formulation of therapy indicates a personal divine mediation in every cure. The god enters personally into the therapeutic effect in each individual case. But when some drug is prescribed there is a new dimension. There arises the significant question, to what extent does essential medicinal virtue lie in the will of the god, to what extent in the prescribed medicine? Certainly, as emphasis rests more and more on drugs, the divine importance tends to recede. Then we have a changing attitude toward disease. When it is the medicine which cures, it is the priest who indicates the medicine while the god merely reveals which medicine is most appropriate for the given case. When the gods played a role secondary to the activity of drugs, when the ability to treat successfully became a function of the priest rather than of the god whom the priest served, then a long step had been taken toward scientific medicine.

Further progress demands a changed attitude toward the patient. Although every individual is unique, the scientific physician recognizes that disease states are not unique. They occur in classes or groups, with common features. Many patients may have the same disease, and a remedy effective for one patient should be effective for another who truly suffers from the same condition. This principle, in a later and more sophisticated dress, became the concept called the uniformity of nature. Without some such understanding there can be no generalization, no learning from experience. When priests applied the lessons learned from one patient to the treatment of a similar patient, they were giving up the religious approach, for they were revising the idea of a unique relationship between the suppliant patient and the healing god. Instead there was the recognition of some sort of regularity independent of divine will, a regularity which allowed for generalizations. The conceptual explanation no longer revolved around a personal superhuman agent, but concerned impersonal factors that could be described and that allowed for prediction.

It is important to realize that predictability by itself is no criterion of a scientific attitude. In mythology the soothsayers might tell in advance how the gods would behave. In the *Iliad,* once the proper measures were taken to follow out the priestly advice, the plague did indeed cease,

as had been predicted. But the significant difference between the mythological and the scientific approach lies in
the explanation offered, the mechanism invoked, the basic
attitude toward the universe.

III

It would be wrong to think that a religious formulation
for disease existed for a period of time and then neatly
gave way to a "scientific" formulation. It is not true that
an idea or a system of ideas simply vanishes, to be replaced
by new concepts. On the contrary, systems have inertia
and tend to persist. Alternatives, even when inconsistent
with each other, may coexist. Various currents and streams
can flow side by side, mingling somewhat, but maintaining surprising identity until they finally merge or disap-
pear. Hippocrates and his school may be taken to represent
the scientific medicine which coexisted for a long time
with the religious and magical aspects of Greek thought.[9]
Hippocrates was born in Cos, probably in 460 B.C. The
date of his death, while uncertain, was probably well into
the fourth century. He was a physician who taught medicine as well as practiced. It is known that he was a member of the Asclepiads, the guild of physicians already mentioned, and that he traveled widely in Greece. Both Plato
and Aristotle refer to him, and even in antiquity he en-
joyed a great reputation. There is a very large body of
medical writing under the name of Hippocrates, the so-
called *Corpus Hippocraticum*. Critics agree that this is
definitely not the work of a single person. As Jones declares, "The Hippocratic collection is a medley, with no
inner bond of unison except that all the works are written
in the Ionic dialect and are connected more or less closely
with medicine or one of its allied sciences. There are the
widest possible divergences of style, and the sharpest pos-

sible contradictions in doctrine."[19] The collection probably represents part of the library of the medical school at Cos. Such a library would contain a wide variety of writings, varying in quality as well as in style. Certain of these writings indicate an author of great genius, but others are quite pedestrian. Some works are purely technical, as texts on surgery or anatomy; others represent various lectures, essays, treatises, case reports, "aphorisms," and precepts; some are designed for physicians, others for students, others for laymen. Stylistic analysis suggests that at least one hundred and fifty years and possibly considerably more separate the earliest from the latest writings. It is generally believed that in the third or second centuries B.C. scholars at the Alexandrian library compiled and edited the writings, but nevertheless there is no single order or arrangement in the various extant manuscripts.

Instead of referring to the single figure of Hippocrates, it might be preferable to use a blanket term, such as the "school of Hippocrates." In this study we are concerned not with the contribution of any single person, but rather with the manifestations of scientific method in those medical writings attributed to Hippocrates. These writings in their totality exhibit many features characteristic of medical science at its best. As has been pointed out, the different texts by no means exhibit a unified point of view. We find various degrees of accuracy in the observations and different degrees of inferential superstructure built upon these observations. Dependence principally on observation indicates so-called empiricism, while extensive elaboration through inference and theory characterizes the rationalistic approach. The Hippocratic writings include straightforward description, simple inferences, broad generalizations and complex theories, thus encompassing all phases of scientific progress. With diverse orientations individual books vary greatly in their degree of empiricism and rationalism, as well as of critical acumen.

The basis of all science is description. The scientist must first of all be an accurate observer, able to describe what he sees and to make his description meaningful for others. What a competent observer narrates as his own experience is often called a "fact." An alleged fact is always subject to correction by other observers, and if others can make the same or closely similar observations, the fact is accepted. Physicians who make lucid and accurate descriptions of fact are highly esteemed. The greatest compliment posterity could pay the English physician Thomas Sydenham was to call him the English Hippocrates.

In the Hippocratic writings there are narrations or case histories that are models of simple direct description. It is worth while quoting one of these case reports:

The wife of Dromeades, having given birth to a daughter and progressing in all other respects normally, was seized by rigors on the second day, accompanied with high fever.

A pain started on the subsequent day in the hypochondrium; nausea and shivering supervened. She did not sleep on succeeding days and was distraught. Breathing deep and slow. . . .

On the second day after the rigors, her stools were normal; the urine thick, white and cloudy . . . no sediment was formed. She did not sleep at night.

Third day . . . generalized cold sweats. . . .

Fourth day. . . . Fell into a stupor. . . . Tongue dry, thirst. Urine little, thin and oily. . . .

Early on the sixth day she suffered from rigors followed quickly by fever and generalized sweating; the extremities were cold and she was delirious with a slow rate of breathing. After a little while convulsions supervened starting in the head and death soon followed.[11]

This is a straightforward narrative, so precise that today, some 2,400 years later, we have no difficulty in making a diagnosis. It is worth noting that the writer was not trying to analyze or to draw conclusions. He merely narrated the course of a particular sick patient without any interpretation, generalization or theory, yet he included enough facts to delineate a pattern of disease, that is, to indicate a "disease entity" which we can identify today. It is unusual to maintain a narrative that is so purely descriptive, so free of subjective interpretation and so accurate.

The observant physician will not rest content merely to observe what is directly before him, but he will look around and deliberately search for connections between various observations. In so doing he is making an interpretation, and he asserts a "belonging together" of various data in a causal relationship. Sometimes the assertions of connection may be quite trivial. For example, in one case report we find the statement that a certain woman "took a high fever with shivering as the result of grief"; or that a young man suffering from shivering, nausea, and insomnia "had been running a temperature for a long time as a result of drinking and much sexual indulgence."[12] These are causal interpretations of individual cases, with no attempt at generality. They assert only that in one particular case a fever was causally related to severe grief, and in another case to lechery. These are inferences (which today we cannot accept) on a simple empirical level.

At other times the inferences may involve acute generalizations, which from the logical standpoint may still be simple and empirical. They may be accurate, yet offer no explanation, no elaboration, no theoretical doctrine. Perhaps the best example of this empirical attitude is the *Prognosis* which scholars universally accept as one of the "genuine" writings of Hippocrates. The ancient Greeks, limited in their therapy, recognized that the important problem was whether the patient would recover or whether he would die. If he were going to die, if treatment would be of no avail, a precise diagnosis did not make very much difference. It was considered more important to know what would happen in the course of the illness, than to have elaborate explanations.

Through careful observations, Hippocrates identified certain broad patterns of recovery, and distinguished those from others, equally broad, in which the patient would die. A correlation was asserted between certain findings that could readily be observed, and death. Or contrariwise, recovery. Perhaps the most famous example is the description of the so-called "Hippocratic facies." Thus, in the seriously ill patient, if we find ". . . the nose sharp, the eyes sunken, the temples fallen in, the ears cold and drawn in and their lobes distorted, the skin of the face hard, stretched and dry, and the colour of the face pale or dusky . . . if there is no improvement, . . . this sign portends death."[13] Or again, "If the hands are waved in front of the face, or make grabs at the air, or pull the nap off cloth, or pull off bits of wool, or tear pieces of straw out of the wall," it is a sign portending death.[14] In view of these quotations it is well to point out how Shakespeare borrowed from Hippocrates when describing the death of Falstaff: ". . . a parted ev'n just between twelve and one, ev'n at the turning o' th' tide: for after I saw him fumble with the sheets, and play with flowers, and smile upon his finger's end, I knew there was but one way; for his nose was as sharp as a pen and a babbled of green fields. . . ."[15]

In the *Aphorisms* and the *Prognostics,* we find abundant correlations of comparable nature. "If the breasts of a pregnant woman regress suddenly, it means that she will have a miscarriage."[16] "Menstrual bleeding which occurs during pregnancy indicates an unhealthy fetus."[17] Or, "Fits or tetanus complicating severe burns are bad."[18] If the bowel movements are very watery or white, it is bad.

Acute earache with continuous severe fever is bad, but if white pus flows from the ear, the patient may recover.[19]

These all represent correlated observations, asserting that certain observed sequences are somehow connected. Experience had shown that if a pregnant woman starts to bleed early in pregnancy it is unlikely that a healthy baby will be born. It was not necessary to mention individual cases, nor considered important to give reasons. But numerous individual observations were summarized in a single pithy statement. Many of these assertions we can wholeheartedly accept today, for the correlations have stood the test of time. Of course, not all the statements are now considered acceptable. When the author declared that "people who lisp are especially liable to prolonged diarrhea,"[20] we refuse to accept the inference, and we declare the statement erroneous.

We must emphasize that the high degree of self-consciousness now prevailing today among scientists is a relatively recent development. The deliberate examination of sources of error, use of controls and statistical techniques, are modern refinements in scientific method which in ancient Greece simply were not part of the medical environment. In the *Aphorisms,* for example, the evidence behind the statement is not given. It might be of some interest to know how many cases of lisping the author saw, how many cases of diarrhea, how uniform was the series of cases, but even if we knew all this, it would not be very helpful. Even with the modern concepts of controls and evaluation of evidence, we find that many assertions made today in good faith turn out to be erroneous. The startling feature, for the modern reader, is not the errors but the amazing insight into medical phenomena and the careful observation displayed in the Hippocratic corpus.

A distinction between observation and inference, between empiricism and rationalism, is basically artificial, since neither can exist without a substantial share of the other. But there can exist a difference in attitude. This, in simplified form, we can indicate by a query. If we challenge a statement and ask the author, "How do you know?" the empiricist will answer, "I saw it." The rationalist will declare, "I figured it out." In almost every statement some observation and some inference are involved, but there can be a difference in proportion. The greater the direct observational component, the greater the empiricism. The further we get from direct observation, the more we depend on inference and reasoning; the more abstract and general our discussion becomes, the greater the rationalism. For science to progress beyond the more elemental stages, some degree of rational approach must be superimposed. Straightforward description, simple correlations and generalizations, express the empirical outlook. As the generalizations become more broad, as explanation supplements description, and as broad general principles are enunciated, we encounter the rationalistic approach.

The Hippocratic writings exhibit all gradations. Let us examine some of the rationalistic components, wherein the place of inference becomes more and more important. One of the Hippocratic writings which stresses the rationalistic approach is *The Science of Medicine,* where we find the distinction between *external* diseases and *internal* diseases. To our modern viewpoint the distinction is scarcely tenable, but the Hippocratic author was expressing an important point, that some changes, such as occurred on the surface of the body, were quite readily and directly observed. They could be noted by the corporeal eye. On the other hand, what takes place in the internal organs could not be directly observed. However, this did not mean we must remain in ignorance. What we cannot see directly with the corporeal eye, we may yet be able to perceive indirectly, by the eye of reason. "What

23

escapes our vision we must grasp by mental sight," and the physician must have recourse to reasoning.[21] That is, what he cannot observe directly he must infer. Indirect evidence and reasoning supplement the direct evidence of the senses.

Indirect evidence is rarely intrusive but must be sought out. The physician, by interrogating the patient, and listening to recital of symptoms, may learn a great deal about the disease. Or the physician may make his observations ". . . on the quality of the voice, whether it be clear or hoarse, on the respiratory rate, whether it be quickened or slowed, and on the constitution of the various fluids which flow from the orifices of the body, taking into account their smell and colour, as well as their thinness or viscosity. By weighing up the significance of these various signs it is possible to deduce of what disease they are the result, what has happened in the past and to prognosticate the future course of the malady."[22] By paying attention to *signs* the physician may be able to build up a picture of the *thing signified,* and reason out or deduce what is the disease.

The signs themselves may not be obvious but may need to be elicited. If the patient cannot cough up anything, certain medicines may bring up phlegm, which can then be inspected. Or, exercise may induce in the respiration certain changes which were not apparent at rest. And through medicine the physician may promote various excretions the better to indicate the disease.[23] It is quite interesting to note how well appreciated was the principle of the functional test, designed to indicate in indirect fashion the status of the internal organs.

The eye of reason may be very important in studying the individual patient. It is even more important, although in a somewhat different way, as the field of inquiry grows. When the scientist wishes to make broad generalizations about whole areas, or whole groups of people, he must necessarily rely more on inference. Although he bases his conclusions on evidence, he must go far beyond literal observation. In some of the Hippocratic writings we have excellent examples of descriptive generalizations in which hypothetical reasoning, dogmatic explanations, and covert inference are heavily incorporated, and mingle diffusely with the elements that are purely descriptive.

In the great text *Airs, Waters, Places,* Hippocrates correlated many diseases with climate, geographical factors, water, and bodily habitus, as well as the prevailing winds. For example, he gave clear objective descriptions of chronic malaria, a condition he associated with stagnant water in marshes and lakes. This general correlation is acceptable and valid. But he intercalated many other inferences and explanations.

Stagnant water from marshes . . . will necessarily be warm, thick and of an unpleasant smell in summer. Because such water is still and fed by rains, it is evaporated by the hot sun. Thus it is coloured, harmful and bilious-looking. In winter it will be cold, icy and muddied by melting snow and ice. This makes it productive of phlegm and hoarseness. Those who drink it have large and firm spleens . . . their faces are thin too because their spleens dissolve their flesh. . . . Their spleens remain enlarged summer and winter and, in addition, cases of dropsy are frequent and fatal to a high degree. The reason for this is the occurrence during the summer, of much dysentery and diarrhoea together with prolonged quartan fevers. Such diseases . . . cause dropsy.[24]

Evaporation by the hot sun he alleged to be a reason for the harmfulness of the water. The water, when cold and muddied, he asserted to be productive of phlegm. Drinking of such water was the cause of the large spleens. It is important to appreciate that although he was wrong, his reasoning was in large part correct. The stagnant water was a fact. It is true that the water was evaporated by the sun. It is true that many people who drank the water contracted malaria, and also diarrhea and dropsy. Therefore he concluded that the water was the cause. He did not distinguish water as something to drink from water as a breeding place for anopheles mosquitoes. He was wrong not because his reasoning was bad but because he lacked detailed knowledge on a descriptive level, and lacked the means of obtaining that knowledge. He put together, as correlates, data which we know did not belong together. He could not discriminate. Progress in medical science is progress in discrimination: as discrimination increases, our inferences and our explanations can become more precise.

Quite different is the error in the following aphorism: "When abnormally fat women do not conceive, it is because the omentum is pressing on the mouth of the womb."[25] Actually he is making two distinct statements; first, that abnormally fat women do not readily conceive, a correlation between marked obesity and infertility that is still approximately valid. The second statement declares a reason for the condition, namely, a mechanical blocking of the mouth of the womb by the omentum. Here we have, as a reason, an alleged fact and an alleged relationship. Both allegations are incorrect. It is patently untrue that the omentum blocks up the uterine opening. A careful observer would have avoided the error, for the means of discrimination were at hand. And a careful scientist would not have offered an explanation that had no factual foundation.

Hippocrates appreciated that causal factors might be complex and peculiarly interrelated. He described[26] a Scythian tribe who were relatively infertile. To explain this he invoked a number of factors. The tribe was nomadic and the men did a great deal of horseback riding, while the women lived in wagons. They inhabited a rather barren territory, in a cold, damp, wintry climate that remained quite uniform all year round. The people, both men and women, were flabby and stout and lacked body hair. Many of the men were impotent, many women sterile. These data can all be accepted as facts. Hippocrates tried to explain the general infertility of the Scythians in the following fashion: *Because* the climate is uniform, without much variation, the bodies are fleshy, soft, moist, and watery. The children sit around too much, which intensifies the fatness. The men and women cannot be prolific *because* they have such a watery constitution. Furthermore, the men are so worn out with horseback riding that *therefore* they are sexually weak. The fat women are sterile *because* the mouth of the womb is sealed over by fat. Additional evidence we would call "controls." Thus, the female servants, who, unlike their mistresses, have a lean sturdy physique, readily became pregnant. Even to our critical sense, this would suggest that the body-type was related to fertility. And as for controls among the men, it is the richest, who ride the most, who suffer especially from impotence, whereas the poor suffer less *because* they do not ride.

There was thus a complex and interlocking series of inferences, which correlated physical constitution with environmental factors, infertility with physical habitus. The work is a masterpiece of thoughtful observation and deliberate reflection. It is not very important that most of it is wrong by today's standards.

IV

The examples so far offered have asserted correlations between observed data, but have all been on a level of concrete immediacy. The concept of the humors, however, embodies much more abstraction and hypothesis. It involves direct observation but has erected a complicated inferential superstructure upon the factual basis.

The humoral theory holds, essentially, that disease states depend on changes in the fluid components of the body. The solid portions might also undergo changes—ulcers and tumors, for example, were all too apparent—but these would be secondary to alterations in the basic fluids. Knowledge of organ function was slender, opportunities for examination infrequent, and interest not very great. There were no adequate means for discriminating the organ changes and hence their causal importance in disease could not be estimated. On the other hand the body fluids were much more readily observed, their changes in quantity or quality relatively apparent and more easily appreciated.

The common cold is a fine example. Normally there is a very slight amount of moisture in the nose. When we have a cold, this amount vastly increases and, as Hippocrates pointed out, the nose swells, becomes hot and inflamed. This change in the nose itself he attributed to an "acrid" quality in the mucus. There could also be a fever. "When the discharge becomes thicker, less acrid, milder and more of its ordinary consistency," the fever falls.[27] As the humors return to their normal state, the patient recovers. Since the nose is no longer so red, he assumed that the mucus was less irritating. Many other diseases showed comparable discharge involving, for example, the eyes, or throat, or lungs. A humor such as phlegm varied in appearance as the disease progressed. Sputum, for example, obviously changed greatly as a bronchitis or a pneumonia ran its course, and there was a fair correlation between the appearance of the sputum and the clinical stage of the disease. We would say that as the patient recovered, the humors returned to normal, but Hippocrates reversed the

28

emphasis: as the humors returned to normal, the patient recovered. He maintained that the discharges became "digested" or underwent "coction," whereby they lost their crude irritating properties and returned to normal. Recovery was consequent upon this coction.

Many diseases revealed great changes in the body fluids. Apart from increased nasal secretions or sputum there were ascites and edema ("dropsy"); vomitus of varying character and dysentery of various types; there were jaundice and vascular congestion and hemorrhages; hydrocephalus and effusion into joints and hydrocele; there were inflammations and discharging wounds, collections of pus and weeping ulcers. All these represented body fluids variously changed from the normal.

As is well known, Hippocrates maintained that there were four humors—the blood, phlegm, yellow bile, and black bile.[28] In more recent times, through the eighteenth century, a great many other body fluids, such as milk, sweat, saliva, earwax, semen, and the like, were explicitly designated as humors. But in Greek thought the number four was somehow especially significant. The primary elements, so-called, were four in number—earth, air, fire, and water; the primary qualities—hot, cold, moist, and dry— were similarly four; Alcmaeon held to the four regions of the body—the head, heart, navel, and pubic region;[29] Aristotle described four causes, and Hippocrates before him held to the four humors; and to these corresponded the four temperaments. If we have an initial prejudice favoring the number four, then any multiplicity greater than that must be reduced to this number. It was quite evident that a single humor can assume many forms. Nasal mucus can be watery and transparent, or thickened and colored, or dried and hard, all these in various degrees. Bile can vary greatly in color, from "white" to very dark green, and in consistency from watery to ropy. Since a single substance can appear under many different forms and still maintain its identity, it was entirely reasonable to hold that cerebro-spinal fluid, nasal mucus, edema fluid, joint effusion, and some types of vomitus or diarrhea, could all represent different forms of the single humor, phlegm. There were no available means for discrimination.

However, a Hippocratic writer strongly combated the monistic view which claimed that the body was composed essentially of a single substance, which underwent various transformations under different conditions. His theory was that the four humors were distinct, different one from the other, and quite irreducible.[30] Nevertheless, one humor could preponderate at a given time. In winter there was the most phlegm, and at this season occurred most of the nasal discharges and sputa. In spring, while phlegm still remained abundant, the quantity of blood increased progressively into the summer. These were the periods when patients had nosebleeds and dysentery ("bloody flux," indicating an excess of blood which passes off through the bowels). During the summer, which is dry and warm, phlegm (whose nature is cold and wet) was at its weakest. During the summer and autumn, he declared, the quantity of bile increased, and this was the season when patients vomited the most bile. The black bile was preponderant in autumn, and "the blood in the body reaches its lowest level in autumn, because this is a dry season and the body is already beginning to cool. . . . And just as the year is governed at one time by winter, then by spring, then by summer and then by autumn; so at one time in the body phlegm preponderates, at another time blood, at another time yellow bile and this is followed by the preponderance of black bile."[31]

To explain disease, physicians elaborated these basic ideas and in so doing drew upon the general cultural her-

itage. The Greeks were devoted to the concept that a due
and proper proportion—the mean—was the standard of
excellence. This was explicitly discussed by both Plato and
Aristotle, but had already formed part of the native tradition. It is only to be expected, therefore, that Hippocratic
physicians leaned upon this concept. Health, it was declared, "is primarily that state in which these constituent
substances are in the correct proportion to each other, both
in strength and quantity, and are well mixed." Pain or
other disturbance resulted when one constituent "presents
either a deficiency or an excess, or is separated in the body
and not mixed with the others."[32] Nature tries to re-estab-
lish the balance of humors. The harmful substances are
rendered innocuous through "coctions" and then eliminated through the vomitus, the sweat, the urine, or sputum, sometimes through hemorrhage or ulcerations or
pus; and then health is re-established, with the humors
once again in the proper proportion.

How do these concepts apply to actual diseases? While
the different Hippocratic treatises are by no means entirely consistent, certain texts offer a fine illustration of the
explanatory process. Phlegm was supposed to arise in the
brain. If during fetal life the brain underwent a normal
development, excess fluid and impurities drained away. If
this occurred to the proper degree, the infant had a perfectly healthy head, but if there were too little "cleansing"
from the fetal brain, this led to a retention of phlegm, and
a phlegmatic constitution necessarily resulted. Excess
phlegm had somehow to be eliminated; otherwise in
later life it might break out in ulcerated sores, excess sali-
vation, or mucus production. Or, if it went to the bowels,
a diarrhea resulted; while if the phlegm "descends cold to
the lungs and to the heart, the blood is chilled," so that
palpitations of the heart and difficulty in breathing en-

sue,[33] not ceasing until the inflowing phlegm had been warmed and dispersed.

Hippocratic views on epilepsy, the "sacred disease," were directly connected with the foregoing doctrines. Epilepsy was considered to have its seat in the brain. It tended to be hereditary and was especially likely to occur in phlegmatic individuals, while those of bilious temperament escaped. The disease arose when the flow of blood to the brain was hindered. The important feature was not the blood itself, but the air or breath, which flowed along in the vessels. If the supply of air was shut off, that is, when veins were ". . . so compressed, when a man is lying or seated, that the breath cannot pass through the vein, a numbness immediately seizes him."[34] (This was his explanation of the familiar "pins and needles" that may result from pressure on a limb.) Now the air, he thought, reached the brain through two major vessels, one coming from the liver, the other from the spleen. If air was prevented from reaching the brain through these vessels, the "sacred disease" resulted.

It was phlegm, coming down from the brain, which was the villain of the piece.[35] We have seen previously that excess phlegm might discharge itself in several different ways. If these various passages were blocked, the excess phlegm might suddenly enter the veins leading to the brain, and shut them off, so that air could not pass. "When the blood-vessels are shut off from this supply of air by the accumulation of phlegm and thus cannot afford it passage, the patient loses his voice and his wits."[36] The Hippocratic text described the epileptic seizure and connected the various aspects thereof with the deprivation of air. "All these symptoms are produced when cold phlegm is discharged into the blood which is warm, so chilling the blood and obstructing its flow."[37] If a great deal of thick phlegm suddenly occluded the vessels, the result was

32

quickly fatal. A lesser quantity, however, might temporarily obstruct and produce symptoms, but the warm blood eventually dispersed the phlegm, the vessels could again admit air, and consciousness returned.

This was indeed a masterly attempt to explain a complex series of phenomena. The phlegm was demonstrably a concrete substance, but to serve as an explanation it had to be endowed with certain hypothetical properties which had not been directly observed. No one saw the phlegm in the brain enter the vessels; no one demonstrated that excess phlegm did in fact shut off air; and although the deprivation of air might induce convulsions (as in asphyxia), no one had demonstrated that epilepsy as a disease was due to the shutting-off of air. The alleged explanation had a certain factual basis but was essentially an imaginative construct. The imagined properties formed a concept which could tie together a great many observations, comparable, as already suggested, to a cord which strings together a mass of beads.

The alleged nature, properties, and relationships of phlegm, therefore, were abstractions, conceptually elaborated. If we could ask a Hippocratic physician how he knew all these things, the answer would be, "I figured it out," or, "It had to be that way." He perceived with the eye of reason. We today would say that the illumination was too dim to allow him to see clearly.

It is quite significant, however, that the explanation was still in terms that were quite close to observation. The various attributed properties and functions were not actually observed but they were all of such a character that they might have been. That is to say, the properties were theoretically observable, and with modern techniques they could be tested experimentally. In other words, although they represented abstractions, they were still in the realm of physics, and relatively close to experience. They were

33

not metaphysical abstractions, but remained in the world of nature. The explanations offered were not in any sense "ultimate." They did not involve metaphysical concepts such as the four elements or the primary qualities or hard little bouncing atoms. The great Hippocratic text *Ancient Medicine* is quite clear that such ultimate explanations are not useful.[38] Hippocrates protested the intrusion of philosophic speculation into medicine, for such speculation is far too abstract to be significant in concrete affairs. It was a great virtue to explain observed sequences in terms that were relatively close to experience and might eventually be tested by further experience.

It is clear that such an attitude is thoroughly scientific, in the most worthy sense. It involves certain postulates that modern writers have made explicit, regarding the so-called uniformity of nature and the idea of "natural law," that what happened once will happen again under the same circumstances. The Hippocratic writers were aware of this. *The Sacred Disease*[39] affirmed the rule of law and natural causation, and expressly denied that the gods played any special role in disease. Superstitions, divine caprice, and chance were rejected. When what we may call "natural law" was considered supreme, then indeed was the foundation of science laid.

V

In some Hippocratic writings there was special concern to show that medicine was truly a science. We note a certain defensive attitude, as if the value of medicine and its claims to scientific status had been impugned and various objections were described in order to be refuted. Some objections sound familiar today. It was claimed that doctors do not agree among themselves and that what one prescribes another considers of no value. This appeared similar to the practice of diviners and augurs, who, from inspection of entrails or observation of omens, would draw quite opposite conclusions.[40] Such disagreement might seem to indicate that the statements were conjecture rather than firm knowledge. Moreover, patients could remain sick despite medical attention, and get well without it. This would suggest that recovery was due to good fortune rather than medical skill.[41]

However, it was the Hippocratic view that medicine is a real science.[42] The very fact that some physicians are effective and others not, that some achieve better results than others, indicates this—"Where there are procedures which can be right or wrong, a consideration of these must constitute a science. I assert that there is no science where there is neither a right way nor a wrong way, but a science consists in the discrimination between different procedures."[43]

This is an assertion of extreme importance. Modern thought would say that there *is* an objective reality which is orderly and which can be observed. This concept the Greeks embodied in their term *physis,* implying that there exists an objective order of things which may be apprehended. There *is* a right way of procedure; or, at least, one mode of doing things is more consonant with the real order, more correct or somehow better, than is another. If there are no means to distinguish the right way from the wrong way, the better from the worse, then we have no objective grounds for our doctrines or our procedure. We then have only chaotic opinion, the negative of science.

Hippocrates was entirely correct when he insisted that science implies a right way and a wrong way, and that there must be some means for deciding which is which. Some criteria must exist, some touchstone, to measure the value, the rightness, of treatment or of theory. What criteria? Hippocrates did not give the answer to this all-

35

important question, but he has the merit of having raised the problem. It is tempting to say that the patient's recovery is the touchstone, but reflection shows that this, while important, is not conclusive. Patients may get well for reasons quite other than the medicines administered, the regimen followed, or the explanations propounded. Hippocrates was quite aware of this.

If we could furnish any really simple means for distinguishing the right procedure or theory from the wrong, for distinguishing truth from error, then all problems would simply melt away. Mankind has long sought some simple criteria. The history of science traces the many different ways whereby man tried to achieve this discrimination, the many ways in which he tried and failed and tried again. Science may be defined as the *search* for the way to discriminate the correct from the incorrect. Hippocrates did indeed give us certain answers. He did indeed achieve a discrimination of a sort. But we cannot accept his answers, for the passage of time has revealed his errors. Nevertheless it was his great virtue to perceive clearly the essential problem and to try hard to achieve a discrimination between the right way and the wrong way in medical science. When we study his writings we gain renewed insight into the nature and methods of science.

The science of medicine depends on the faith that it is not chance which operates, but cause. Since all phenomena will be found to have a cause, and "chance" is no more than an empty name,[44] it follows that those who rightly perceive the causes and act accordingly will be the better practitioners; and, conversely, the better practitioner perceives causes more rightly. The scientific practitioner has as one of his attributes the understanding of causes. Hippocrates held a rather dim view of the abilities of the average practitioner. Most doctors, he declared, were comparable to navigators who appear to do quite well in calm weather, when any mistakes would not be apparent. But in a storm this incompetence becomes evident, and the ship will be lost.[45]

We do not need to labor the point that there are good doctors and bad doctors, for there always have been and presumably always will be. Temkin[46] has emphasized the different classes of medical practitioners in the Greco-Roman world. There were the ordinary practitioners, who learned by rote or apprenticeship, whom Temkin calls "leeches." These would be the lower classes, who might have skill but no theoretical knowledge. There was also the higher class, the physicians who studied nature (*physis*), and who knew the theories and could explain the causes.

The conceptions of medical science which were current in ancient Greece have produced considerable semantic confusion in present-day thinking. The difficulty has revolved around the term *techne,* which has generally been translated as *art,* and which has given rise to a very false distinction between something called the "art of medicine" and something else called the "science of medicine." This, in turn, has produced conflicting imagery, between a warm sympathetic practitioner who may not know very much but who by intuition is able to help his patient; and another figure, cold and aloof, who deals in tests and gadgets. The difficulty is resolved if we examine certain basic meanings that were made very explicit by Aristotle.

He used three separate terms, *empeiria, techne,* and *episteme,* which have usually been translated "experience," "art," and "science." When the meanings are examined, the confusion disappears.

"Experience" refers primarily to the learning process. Something happens to us; we remember it; this memory influences our behavior the next time we meet a similar situation. Through this "learning by experience" we acquire the ordinary skills of life. But man (and according to Aristotle, man alone) not only learns by experience but is capable of reasoning. That is, he can deal in abstractions and generalizations. "Experience" he acquires from individual instances many times repeated, but "reason" passes beyond the individual event. In Aristotle's words, "From many notions of experience a single universal judgment is formed with regard to like objects."[47]

When we abstract, generalize, and deal with universal rules and judgments, we engage in *techne,* whose distinction from *empeiria* is expressed by the English opposition "rational" and "empirical." This distinction is especially clear in medicine, wherein Aristotle's own words are still applicable: "To have a judgment that when Callias was suffering from this or that disease, this or that benefitted him, and similarly with Socrates and various other individuals, is a matter of experience; but to judge that it benefits all persons of a certain type, considered as a class, who suffer from this or that disease . . . this is a matter of art (*techne*)."[48] We cease to act from rule of thumb, and instead act according to general principles.

Techne has been commonly translated by the Latin *ars,* from which, of course, come "art" and "artisan." *Techne,* however, is also the root of "technology" and "technique" and may be rendered "science," as in the most recent translation of Hippocrates, by Chadwick and Mann. "Life is short, science is long,"[49] conveys a quite different English sense from the more familiar translation, "Life is short, art is long." If we wish to equate classical Greek thought with present-day idiom, then *techne* should be rendered as "science."

The man of experience may be distinguished from the man of science, just as today we distinguish an electrician from an electrical engineer. Aristotle contrasted the *cheirotechnes* or handicraftsman who, as the word indi-

cates, worked with his hands, and the *architechton,* the
director or engineer, who worked largely with his head.
These are ordinarily translated "artisan" and "master
craftsman," respectively.[50] The modern distinction might
be that of technician and doctor.

In ancient times medicine was strictly comparable to the
so-called trades, and the physician to the mason, ship-
wright, or navigator. All aimed at achieving some practical end or goal. While these practitioners all could learn
their trade by rule of thumb, and could all improve with
practice, they could also learn theoretical background.
Techne represents this theoretical background, the generalizations, the principles which underlie the practical
activity and which were founded in the nature of things.
To be sure, theoretical knowledge does not of itself make
a man dexterous. The man with only practical experience
—the empiric—may be more successful in getting something done than the theorist without experience. But those
who have knowledge of causes, who understand theory,
are wiser than men who only have experience.[51]

Techne can be taught. It conveys *information about—*
the how and the why, the causes at work, the principles
that operate, the right way and the wrong way, and why
this is so. The good teacher need not be the good per-
former. The golf professional or the operatic coach may
not be the best player or the best singer, but he understands the principles underlying good playing or good
singing. Experience, on the other hand, cannot be taught.
It must be acquired. We can, for example, tell a student
how to perform an appendectomy, but nothing can substitute for his actually doing it.

It is quite in the spirit of Greek thought and at the same
time consonant with modern idiom, to say that *techne*
seeks the regularities in nature, or, in loose phraseology,

the laws which govern phenomena. This is what we mean today by science.

But there is one very important further distinction: that between *techne* and *episteme*. *Techne* indeed seeks the laws which govern phenomena, but only of those phenomena which have some practical application. For Aristotle this included such activities as medicine or architecture or navigation. There are, however, activities which do not seek any practical advantage but are essentially contemplative in nature. These are the realm of *episteme*.

Aristotle sharply distinguished practical knowledge from theoretical, or, as we might say today, applied science from pure science. Practical knowledge aimed at something other than itself, and its object was some sort of activity—*doing* something. Theoretical knowledge aimed only at truth, not practical results.[52] The merely practical has to do with the contingent, which comes into being and passes away, which may be true at one moment but not at another, depending on various factors and events. The rules of medicine, for example, might apply to most patients but not to all. There is the realm of more-or-less, of "maybe" and "it depends." But Aristotle believed there was another kind of knowledge that was true by necessity —eternal, unchangeable, and not capable of being otherwise than it is.[53] The simplest example is mathematics. The propositions of geometry—for example, the truths about squares and triangles and circles—are true by necessity. Characteristic of knowledge of this sort is the certainty with which the conclusions can derive from the initial principles. This is the meaning of the phrase "not capable of being otherwise."

For Aristotle the theoretical or contemplative sciences include mathematics, physics, and theology.[54] Apart from contemplation, there is not much we can *do* about them. We cannot, thought Aristotle, change the properties of

40

triangles or of matter; we cannot change the course of the celestial spheres or the attributes of God. What was detached, impersonal, contemplative, eternally true, and unchangeable, possessed a much higher value than the practical. Translated into modern terms, pure basic science, not concerned with personal advantage or with concrete application or practical benefits, was the highest activity.

We must not, of course, attribute to Hippocratic writers the carefully reasoned assertions of Aristotle. Nevertheless the concept seems implicit, however vaguely, in some Hippocratic writings. Or phrased differently, the philosophy which underlies many Hippocratic writings seems consistent with the philosophy which Aristotle later expressed so clearly.

While we must constantly remember that the various Hippocratic writings do not form a doctrinal unity, and may even contradict one another, yet there is perhaps an over-all trend. This, from a distant perspective, we may try to summarize. Hippocratic medicine was based on careful observation. Events, however, were observed not in isolation but in relation to other events. The physician notes regularities, patterns and relations, and the togetherness of things. The better the physician, the broader the patterns which he distinguishes. There is also the full realization that the patterns and regularities, as well as the seemingly isolated events, represent neither chance nor a capricious personal will. They express the nature of things as they are, the *physis*. The physician learns from experience, but at the same time he seeks knowledge of causes. He must employ not merely his senses but also the eye of reason, to understand the *physis*. He deals in general principles, which must be appropriately applied. But medicine is a practical activity. The knowledge of causes must be relative to the goals of medicine. Hence unbridled speculation, concern with ideas far from immediate experience, are not the province of the physician.

Such a philosophy has a very modern ring, and would be quite applicable in modern times. Perhaps the most recent medical perspectives have changed somewhat. Practical medicine has received unexpected help from the speculations of the mathematicians and the physicists, so much so that modern medicine fully appreciates the essential unity of all the sciences. The *physis* is seen to be far more complex than might have been thought, and the properties of ultimate matter are truly revelant to medical science. If we permit this modification, then the Hippocratic viewpoint would be entirely applicable today.

Sophistication

GALEN, THE "FACULTIES," AND THE "PROBLEM OF CHANGE"

The six centuries that separated Hippocrates from Galen saw a tremendous change in material civilization, social behavior, and cultural environment. The great age of Pericles drew to a close; Greek philosophy reached its unsurpassed heights; the Macedonian empire rose and fell; the Roman republic grew mighty; her foreign wars changed the face of the Western world, while her civil wars led to even more profound internal changes. With the establishment of empire, the Golden Age flowered, gave way to the Silver Age, and then to the long slow decline which contemporary observers could not see. Galen lived in the second century A.D., during the period of Stoic philosophy and early Christianity, of high culture and sophistication, great material achievement and considerable unrest.

The main facts of Galen's life are readily told. Born in Pergamon, in Asia Minor, his birth date is usually given as A.D. 130. Nicon, his father, was an architect, cultured and well educated. Of his mother Galen declared that she was very bad-tempered, often shouting, scolding, and quarreling, and worse than Xantippe, the shrewish wife of Socrates. Heredity may have worked in devious ways, for Galen's writings often seem unduly acrimonious and controversial, perhaps a chromosomal legacy from his mother.

Pergamon, the site of a very famous Aesculapian temple, was a city of outstanding culture. The young Galen, under his father's guidance, received a fine liberal education. Until he was seventeen he studied philosophy with the best masters, preparing for a career in public service. But his father had a dream directing his attention to medicine, the boy concurred, and began his medical studies. For four years longer he remained at Pergamon. Then, when his father died, he furthered his medical education in Smyrna, Corinth, and finally Alexandria, where he stayed for five years. When he was twenty-eight years of age and had devoted eleven years to medical studies, he returned to Pergamon, where he became physician to the gladiators, a position which provided abundant medical and surgical experience. After four years, however, he went to Rome, just when Marcus Aurelius became emperor. The young Greek was very successful professionally, achieving a high reputation as practitioner as well as anatomist. It is said, however, that he aroused the antagonism of many physicians, charlatans, and others. Whether this antagonism drove him out, or whether he fled from an outbreak of the plague, is not clear, but he did leave Rome and returned to Pergamon. However, the emperor ordered him to join the army at Aquileia (near the present Venice), and after a short stay sent him back to Rome, as medical attendant to the prince Commodus. This office he performed for perhaps six years, but continued to live in Rome until about A.D. 192. Then he returned again to Pergamon, where he died in 200.

Galen's voluminous writings covered many fields, including medicine and surgery, anatomy and physiology, materia medica, medical history, and, by no means least, a philosophy of medicine. In his works he strongly opposed any materialistic or atomistic doctrine and condemned narrow mechanistic attitudes. Instead, his viewpoint we may call organismic and purposive: the bodily parts, the whole organism, and the larger environmental whole, exert on each other reciprocal influences, and this interaction involves the concept of *goal* or *purpose*.

His teachings were based partly on evidence and partly on the logical inferences that he could draw therefrom. But Galen blended logic and evidence in a manner not entirely pleasing to us today. He was a keen observer and a good experimentalist, but he pursued logical inferences to a degree that we may consider excessive. He reasoned largely by analogy, a form of logic subject to serious pitfalls. Such an approach allowed him to have a broad synoptic outlook covering a wide range of phenomena, but, while gaining in breadth he often lost depth and accuracy. Nevertheless he observed well, reasoned with great subtlety, paid considerable attention to causation, and demonstrated an advanced degree of scientific methodology. The fact that later ages often proved him wrong does not necessarily detract from the soundness of his method. Instead, his errors furnish us a very valuable workshop for anatomizing the methods of medical science.

Several misconceptions about Galen are firmly fixed in

45

the popular mind. First, he is supposed to have shackled the medical thought of the Middle Ages, exerting a stultifying influence that lasted into the eighteenth century. We can find, for example, an assertion that Galen "endeavored to unite medicine with the metaphysics of Plato. This unfortunate move arrested the further progress of medicine for more than a thousand years."[1] Or, "It was Galen's gratuitous postulation of special forces for each need, even more than his teleology, which risked stopping, *and did stop,* scientific investigations."[2] Or, "He was the prophet of a new kind of dogmatism. For nine centuries he was supreme and alone; then he was joined by the Muslim physician and philosopher Avicenna, and they ruled together until the seventeenth century."[3] Necessarily we must admit that medical progress was relatively slow during the dark ages and the Middle Ages, yet we cannot support the idea that Galen, whatever his errors, was responsible for lack of progress thirty or forty generations after his death.

A second popular condemnation stemmed from Galen's views on movement of the blood. He had asserted that blood passed from the right ventricle to the left, directly through the septum, and that this part of the heart wall contained invisible pores, through which the transfer took place. Popular opinion has often regarded this as sheer imagination, a benighted if not an imbecile error, uncritically accepted until Vesalius, a knight in shining armor, refused assent and inaugurated modern medical science. This view, however, is wrong. Instead, as we shall show, Galen's teachings on the movement of blood were remarkably well reasoned and based on excellent evidence.

Another popular condemnation concerns the so-called "faculties." Perhaps more than any other single feature this doctrine of faculties has tended to throw Galen's system into disrepute. A thing happens, it seems to say, because there is a "faculty" for making it happen. Molière satirized this viewpoint to the ultimate absurdity when he created the immortal "virtus dormativa." In *Le Malade Imaginaire,* we recall, a candidate for the medical degree is asked why opium puts one to sleep. To this the candidate replies that opium acts as it does because it has a soporific faculty. Within the drug is a sleep-making power whose nature it is to deaden the senses. This answer, in Molière's comedy, brought forth the admiring plaudits, "Bene, bene, bene bene respondere." Yet this satire, however appropriate in the seventeenth century, should not be applied to Galen, as we will try to show in a subsequent section. Indeed, all three criticisms we consider to be quite inappropriate, and to reflect certain misconceptions about scientific method and scientific medicine.

To enter sympathetically into Galen's teachings we must appreciate one of his basic principles: everything in nature has its purpose. Nature, he thought, exhibits foresight and skill, and *does nothing in vain.* These propositions which, of course, are not subject to proof, underlie his physiology. Consequently we must begin with the principle that every structure has a function. The structure we can see, the function we can infer. Sometimes, to be sure, function could be directly observed, but usually only with difficulty, for at that time physiological experiments were rather limited in technique and scope. Anatomical structures were much easier to study. From such structures judicious reasoning might lead to the truth regarding function.

But—*was* the reasoning judicious? How can we find out? One test is whether we can support the inferences by appeal to experience. This formula is so popular today that no other mode seems acceptable. But we should be a little more flexible in our thinking, and appreciate the method that Galen most frequently utilized, namely, appeal to analogy. Galen was quick to note similarities between objects, to find common threads and uniformities among things that might appear dissimilar. If he could support an inference by pointing to an analogy, he assumed that his inference was justified. Unfortunately, he did not appreciate the limitations of analogy, namely, that similarities in one aspect may mask very profound differences, so profound that the similarities are actually irrelevant. In such a case we say that the similarities are superficial and the analogy is false. This is a problem in the evaluation of evidence, a problem that is still very far from solution today. An interesting example is Galen's discussion of the function of the omentum, that apron of fat which hangs down in front of the intestines and which, we recall, Hippocrates thought might cover over the neck of the womb to cause sterility (se p. 26). Galen had more advanced notions. He thought the omentum had the function of warming the internal organs.

Now what was the evidence that Galen offered to support his claim? The omentum, he pointed out, was light, firm, and could heat without compressing. (The twentieth century might offer the analogy of an eider-down quilt in winter.) Galen pointed out that the omentum was provided with many blood vessels and much fat. (We can readily appreciate that blood is warm, and we can offer the analogy of an electric blanket, which contains many warm "elements.") And the fat? The fat, Galen pointed out, had an affinity with fire, because it burned easily. His reasoning was that nothing which is "cold"—i.e., contains the elemental quality "cold" to a significant degree—will burn readily. Fat burns readily; therefore it has affinity with elemental heat and may be regarded as intrinsically "hot."

So far Galen had indulged in reasoning. But he gave actual concrete evidence, which might be called controlled observations. He pointed to patients (presumably gladiators) who were wounded, in whom the omentum had to be ablated, and who thus differed from the normal. All such wounded persons, he declared, feel cold in the stomach, digest less well (implying an insufficiency of vital heat, *vide infra*), and require extra covering. He described a particular wounded gladiator who had almost total ablation of the omentum. He healed rapidly but was very sensitive to cold, and could not bear to have his abdomen exposed, always keeping it covered with wool.[4] Such evidence seemed to prove his contention.

Modern criticism could raise two points. One is purely methodological. How many cases did he have? His evidence was statistically insufficient and not "properly" controlled. This same criticism, of course, is very much bandied about today, in regard, say, to the effectiveness of many vaccines, or the causal role of smoking in lung cancer. In the matter of inadequate controls Galen is in excellent company. A second point concerns inadequate knowledge. Galen's cited case is actually irrelevant, for the symptoms he described were those of hyperesthesia. These symptoms presumably stemmed from nerve damage in the abdominal wall and were quite independent of the omentum. However, this he could not possibly know.

While Galen's modes of thought may seem somewhat strange to us, we must preserve a judicious historical attitude. If what our distant or recent ancestors wrote seems silly or foolish to us, we may draw one of (at least) two conclusions: Either they *were* fools, and consequently what they said *was* foolish; or, on the contrary, they *were not* fools, and hence if what they said appears foolish, then we simply do not understand the background against which they moved. The twentieth century does not have any corner on brains. Our ancestors were by and large at least as intelligent as we are. Hence, if anyone whom we consider intelligent makes pronouncements that seem absurd, the fault probably lies with us for not entering sufficiently into his mental state. The historian of ideas should reconstruct a background within which the contemporary statement would seem reasonable. If he does not do this, then the historian may exhibit the sort of condescending attitude which ran through much of nineteenth-century historical writing. We believe that epithets like "foolish," when applied to Galen's doctrine, are entirely inappropriate.[5]

II

The doctrines and methods of Galen may be introduced by consideration of the "invisible pores" which he postulated in the cardiac septum. To appreciate this hypothesis we must understand his doctrine regarding blood and spirits. As is well known, Galen maintained there were three *pneumata* or spirits, the natural, vital, and animal, which presided over various bodily functions. In modern terminology these refer to three major functional areas and indicate divisions still appropriate in physiology: the "vegetative," which covers the most basic functions of digestion, nutrition, excretion, and reproduction; the "cardiovascular" or circulatory aspects; and the "neuromuscular," which serve integration, locomotion, and mental activity. These are all interrelated.

The major sequences of digestion can serve as a starting point. Ingested food is broken down, in many successive steps, within the gastrointestinal tract. The chyle so produced is absorbed into the intestinal veins which pass to the liver. Here the chyle is elaborated into blood and endowed with the vegetative or "natural" spirits. Galen was a humoralist, as was Hippocrates; he could readily observe and appreciate the variations in body fluids. It was apparent that somehow the solid organs "acted on" the fluids, but just how was not at all clear. The specific differences between the various solid organs could not be readily observed. At best the functions could be inferred. That chyle became transformed into blood within the liver was such an inference. It was a fact of observation, however, that blood from the liver entered the great veins.

And what about the arteries? Their function was not clear. The earlier viewpoint, which Galen combated, was that of Erasistratus, who maintained that while the veins carried blood, the arteries carried air (pneuma) which had entered the lungs and thence passed to the left heart by the pulmonary veins.* From the left heart, Erasistratus thought, the air passed to the aorta and its arterial branches. These arteries after death contained air, not fluid. If during life a severed artery yielded blood, this fact could readily be explained. When an artery was severed, an instantaneous escape of pneuma could be assumed. This escape created a vacuum, which then sucked blood out of the veins,[6] rather as in a siphoning process.

Galen, however, would not accept all this. He knew that arteries carried blood, and his demonstration of this fact was a very important contribution. Furthermore, he was well acquainted with the cardiac valves and their function.[7] He knew that there were communications between the arteries and veins;[8] that inspired air was necessary for life; that waste products had to be removed in respiration; and that the pneuma concerned the lungs, the heart, and the blood. The relationships among all these factors were quite complex and not always consistently

---

* In this discussion I use modern terminology. The older terms, "vein-like artery" and "artery-like vein," can be very confusing to the unwary. They emphasize that all vessels to or from the right heart were considered veins, all those on the left, arteries. But otherwise the terms serve no useful purpose today.

described. Recent authors[9] have indicated that some time-honored interpretations, expressed by many prominent medical historians seriatim, do not accurately reflect Galen's thought.

Respiration, the inflow and outflow of air, took place for the sake of the "innate heat."[10] Galen compared the innate heat in the heart to a lamp which was burning; a lamp requires air in order to burn and also requires removal of sooty wastes, lest it smother.[11] Inspired air, then, which entered the lungs, performed a cooling and ventilating function. It passed to the heart by the pulmonary veins, and most of it passed back to the lungs by the same veins,[12] carrying with it the sooty vapors. For this to occur there had to be some reflux from the left ventricle, retrograde against the mitral valve.[13] It follows that the waste material from the heart was yielded up from the left ventricle, not from the right.

Now the role of the blood in all this is quite clear. There were two sorts of blood, that in the veins and that in the arteries. The venous blood was darker and exhibited a to-and-fro movement that should not, however, be construed as necessarily regular or rhythmic. The arterial blood was lighter and hotter, and was propelled by pulses which originated in the heart. Why should there be two kinds of blood? It was Nature's provision that some bodily parts "should be nourished by pure, thin and vaporous blood, and others by thick turbid blood."[14] The arterial blood, which was thinner and more vaporous, contained pneuma. Galen suggested that some pneuma in the arterial blood came from the lungs.[15] But he also thought that the arteries could communicate with the skin through which they could draw in air. Thus, of the arteries he said, "Just as through the mouths terminating in the skin they excrete all such vapors or smoky stuff they have. Or they take up not a little portion from the surrounding air into

52

themselves."[16] Or again, "Those arteries which reach the skin draw in the outer air when they dilate."[17] The arterial blood contains, then, some vivifying principle which the venous blood does not have.

But, wherever and however the pneuma enters the blood, there remains the important problem, *Where does the arterial blood itself come from?* Erasistratus, of course, who believed the arteries contained air, did not have to face any such problem, but for Galen it was inescapable. All blood was formed in the liver, and passed into the vena cava, and thus was carried to the right heart. But then what? To be sure, from the right heart there arose an efferent vessel, the pulmonary artery, which carried blood to the lungs. But this had for its purpose the nourishment of the lungs.[18] How the blood got into the left ventricle was not at all apparent. To us, in the era following Harvey, it all seems so simple. But the problem is very difficult *if we assume that the blood does not circulate.* If we make such an assumption, then Galen's reasoning appears very sound. We may indicate several logical steps.

(1) Blood arising in the liver reaches the right ventricle. (2) Some of this blood goes to the lungs through the pulmonary artery. (3) But the size of the afferent vessels (venae cavae) is greater than the outgoing vessel (pulmonary artery),[19] indicating that more blood is brought into the right ventricle than leaves it through the pulmonary artery.[20] (4) The right side of the cardiac septum shows, as facts of observation, "a kind of fossae with wide mouths, and they get constantly narrower; it is not possible, however, actually to observe their extreme terminations, owing both to the smallness of these and to the fact that when the animal is dead all the parts are chilled and shrunken."[21] (5) Nature does nothing in vain, but all structures have functions. (6) The eye of reason can discern truths which the physical eye cannot perceive.

53

All these propositions are eminently reasonable. They all derive from observation. They cannot be called figments of imagination. Instead, given this set of premises, the conclusion is virtually inescapable, that blood passes from the right ventricle, through the pits in the septum, into the left ventricle. And clearly, from the left ventricle it moves through the aorta into the smaller arteries.

Unfortunately, Galen did not distinguish adequately between what he saw with the corporeal eye and what he saw with the eye of reason. This failure was a major defect in his scientific method. As a scientist he fully appreciated the significance of *facts,* that is, concrete objects of sensory observation. But as a scientist he also realized that facts by themselves are quite sterile. To be fruitful they must point beyond themselves, and must lead to inferences and generalizations. A philosophic tradition going back to Plato and Pythagoras maintained that the "senses" can at best achieve only an approximation, while "reason" can achieve the truth. Hence, somehow, a generalization might be construed as more valuable and closer to truth than the perception from which the inferences arose. This is, of course, very often the case, but not always. Some inferences are valid, some partly valid, some quite invalid. How to tell which is which?

No formula can be given, no set of rules drawn up, which will answer this question. The answer depends on something we can only designate "critical judgment." It is true that modern scientific method has developed certain techniques for checking validity, techniques which involve statistics and controls. But statistics are not the substitute for critical judgment. There is much truth in the well-known quip that figures do not lie but liars do figure. There were critical investigators before these various techniques were developed, and uncritical investigators after they were common property. As for Galen, we will see that he appreciated the difference between sound and faulty inferences in many cases but not in all. Like so many scientists, he was critical but not critical enough.

It is quite surprising how many errors arise because an investigator did not ask the "right" questions. We can say this only after the fact, that is, after someone else came along who *did* ask certain particular questions. Then we realize how errors could have been avoided had these questions only been asked earlier. Galen's views on the heart are a case in point. For example, had he asked himself the question, *Do* the pulmonary veins really contain air, as theory indicates? he would undoubtedly have anticipated Harvey. His reasoning demanded that these veins transport air. If he realized that they were full of blood, he might have revised his theory. But apparently he never asked the question and so never sought a direct answer.

Galen certainly knew that the arteries and veins anastomose, not only in the lungs but peripherally.[22] He knew that under certain circumstances the blood could pass from one set of vessels to the other, but he did not maintain that these connections played any significant role. Of course, he did not *see* the connections, whose existence he merely inferred. For example, a severed artery will drain the blood from the veins.[23] Such an observation entailed, as a logical and necessary consequence, a connection between the two sets of vessels. But having asserted this connection, which he perceived with the eye of reason, he did not ask further questions which might have been relevant.

It is very significant that Galen did not ask questions which involved quantity.[24] Harvey, on the other hand, did. Harvey wanted to know "How much?" *How much* blood was pumped in an hour? Where did all this *quantity* of blood come from? If he had not had this interest in quantitative problems, Harvey would not have discerned the circulation. Galen, on the other hand, had little interest in quantitative relationships. Galenic medicine may be described as a qualitative approach to reality. Such an attitude asks different questions, achieves different formulations, from those dictated by quantitative interests. It is, however, profound error to hold that all science must necessarily be quantitative, or, what comes to the same thing, that unless investigation is quantitative, it is not science.

III

The Galenic "faculties" are much more easily understood if we appreciate certain of the Greek philosophic speculations. Biology is necessarily concerned with the problem of change, that is, with the question, In the ceaseless change around us, what, if anything, remains permanent? Things come into being, and then pass away. There are movement and transition, increase and diminution. Wheat becomes flour. Flour and water turn into bread. Bread and meat become flesh and bone, but these eventually decay and disintegrate. Everything appears to be in flux. Is there anything which remains stable, regardless of how the external appearances may alter? And if there is anything which endures, how can we explain the various transformations which take place?

This, in brief, represents the so-called problem of change, which has intrigued philosophers from earliest times, and which is still very real and important, pursuing us wherever we go, if only we notice it. In the nursery, the child plays with blocks and builds a wall. He knocks it over and the wall is gone. It has disappeared. But the blocks out of which it was made still remain as relatively permanent elements from which the child can make a new structure. In time, however, the blocks can become chipped and broken and quite useless. Yet although these blocks may lose their identity, the wood or plastic from which they were made still persists as relatively permanent.

If we continue the analytic process, we can ask, What is wood made of? What persists if the wood is, say, burned? But then, although we can give a pat answer and talk glibly of molecules, we get into some difficulty. We are leaving the world of everyday observation, of material things we can readily see and handle, and are passing into a much more shadowy world of concepts and hypotheses.

The ancient Greeks had already entered that world and had provided a number of different answers to the problem of change. Observing the flux around them and reflecting on its deeper nature, the early Greek thinkers initiated both science and philosophy. We wish to stress the essential unity of these subjects. The early scientists were the early philosophers, and the converse is equally true.

Thales of Miletus (640–546 B.C.) is generally considered the first who not only asked the question, What is the world made of? but gave a reasoned answer based on observation. He believed that the basic substance was water, which can exist in a variety of forms, such as solid, liquid, or gas, and still maintain its identity. Thales thus indicated a very important principle, that a substance can change its characteristics very markedly and yet remain the same. Conversely, materials of widely different appearance and properties can nevertheless be essentially one, identical in essence and *real* nature, even though not in outward form.

While Thales stressed the inner reality rather than the outward appearance, his conclusions quite outran his evidence. If we assert that there is one basic substance, and if we identify this with some known entity such as water, then we face the problem, How does anything else, like

57

wood or stone, or animals, arise? If everything is *really* water, how does it happen that so many things appear to be not-water? If there is an underlying unity, whence does diversity arise? A brilliant answer was offered by another Miletan philosopher, Anaximenes, who thought that air was the principal substance. Diversity he explained through rarefaction or condensation of the one single element. Thus, Anaximenes said of air, "When it is dilated so as to be rarer, it becomes fire; while winds, on the other hand, are condensed air. Cloud is formed from air by felting; and this, still further condensed, becomes water. Water, condensed still more, turns to earth; and when condensed as much as it can be, to stones."[25]

This is a very important landmark in thought, indicating as it did a quantitative structure to the world, that is, one basic material which is subject to quantitative variations. The diversity of things Anaximenes explained by invoking *more* or *less* of the basic material. This, he thought, accounted for the observed differences between one object and another. Such a concept allowed much greater flexibility in explaining phenomena.

The concept of one basic substance—a simple monistic doctrine—led to contradiction. The alternate doctrine is some sort of pluralism, that is, the view that the ultimate forms of existence are multiple, not single. Certain pluralist doctrines are especially significant for medical theory. To understand Galen we should consider briefly three key figures and their teachings.

Empedocles (500?–430? B.C.) was a physician who, it is worth noting, not only was a philosopher but also founded a school of medicine. He wrote in verse, and only fragments have come down to us. Interpretation is admittedly difficult.

He made explicit the influential doctrine of the four elements, usually called fire, air, earth, water, but sometimes sun, sky, earth, and sea. The substances were homogeneous, indestructible, unchangeable—in other words, true *elements*. Instead of monism with its single element there were now four elements, each with its own qualities, that is, a true pluralism. Any material object, he believed, was composed of the primitive elements combined in various proportions. Thus, bones were four parts of fire, two of earth, and two of water, while in blood the components were mingled in equal proportion. We do not know the evidence on which he based these pronouncements. But he did indicate that material objects in the world around us exhibited both qualitative and quantitative variation. Objects were composed of qualitatively different elements, combined in different proportions. Empedocles maintained two different principles, quality and quantity, as basic explanations of the world around us.

Not content with a bare static analysis, Empedocles provided some sort of dynamic approach. Mere elements by themselves, he thought, would be inert. They required some motive power, some *force* at work. In order to explain motion or activity he invoked two elemental forces, which he called Love and Strife, the one making for harmony and attraction of opposites, the other for discord and separation of opposites. Apparently he considered Love and Strife somehow as material particles, but in their functions as force they provided the kinetic and dynamic factor necessary to activate the other elements.

Empedocles provided a systematic framework for understanding the world. He recognized distinct irreducible elements, he appreciated the quantitative aspects of reality, and he invoked special dynamism or motive power, distinct from the other elements. The concept of the "four elements," variously modified, was very influential throughout ancient and medieval times, and even well into the Renaissance. Empedocles held that these elements

59

cannot be transformed one into the other. What appears to us to be change or transition is only the rearrangement of what permanently exists—"a mingling and a divorce of what has been mingled."[26] Or, in Burnet's translation, "There is no coming into being of aught that perishes . . . but only mingling and change of what has been mingled."[27]

This formulation had certain drawbacks. It did not adequately account for the richly varied *qualities* that exist around us. The actual properties of things, what we actually see and smell and touch—how did they arise out of four material elements, even when distributed in different proportions? An ingenious solution was offered by Anaxagoras (500?–428 B.C.). Unfortunately the textual fragments that have come down to us are at many crucial points very obscure, and interpretation of his doctrine is by no means univocal. In the present account I rely especially on Bailey,[28] who gives a carefully reasoned discussion of controversial points; and also on Aristotle's extended comments.[29]

Let us, by way of understanding Anaxagoras, examine a piece of bread. We find that no matter how much we crumble it or subdivide it, it nevertheless remains bread, with all bread's characteristic qualities. But if we eat it, then the bread becomes flesh and blood. There has occurred what seems at first glance to be a complete transformation. To explain how one object can turn into something else entirely different, Anaxagoras said that the blood and flesh *were present in the bread all the time*. It is not possible for flesh to be created out of not-flesh. When we derive nourishment from food, "the only explanation of the phenomenon is that hair and flesh and the rest must already have been present in the food."[30] This doctrine he generalized, to the extent of saying that there was "a portion of everything in everything."

60

This means that any object must have within it the
seeds or particles of everything that it can ever become.
Since any object may undergo changes quite without
limit, then any object must have within itself an unlimited
number of small particles or seeds, each having the *quality*
which will eventually become manifest. The wheat must
have within itself the quality of bread, which encloses the
quality of flesh, but in addition has multiple other qualities
associated with wheat or bread or flesh. Any individual
object, then, embodies an unlimited number of *qualitatively different* seeds. These seeds are not of any determinate size, for then any object could contain only a finite
limited number. They could be infinitely small. Anaxagoras held specifically that there was no limit to the process
of division, no limit to the number of seeds. There is
some of everything in everything.

It follows that instead of only four elements there is
actually an infinite profusion of elements, all qualitatively
different. No longer is there any difficulty in accounting
for the qualitative variety of the world, for all the elements out of which things are made are *qualities,* which
can combine and recombine but cannot be destroyed. But
Anaxagoras encountered difficulties. If there is some of
everything in everything, why does any particular object
have its own determinate character? If bread contains
seeds of everything, why does it look like bread? The answer is, that the object takes the form of those particles
which predominate. "It is quite true that bread contains
. . . portions of everything, but because the portions of
bread greatly exceed in number and bulk those of any
other thing, it has throughout the appearance and character of bread and nothing else. The subordinate portions
. . . which bread may become, are so minute and so scat-
tered in among the prevailing portions of bread, that they
not merely are not perceived, but never could be percep-

tible . . . they are in fact . . . only 'perceptible in thought.' "[31]

The component seeds, representing a fusion of all things, differ one from the other according to the dominant quality. "There would thus be a 'gold-seed,' for instance, containing the fusion of all things, but dominated by the presence of gold, a 'bone-seed' in which bone was the ascendant. . . . And in this difference of character between seed and seed lies the explanation of the phenomena of change."[32] The latent seeds, as, for example, the flesh- or bone-seeds present in bread, become separated out in digestion and, joining the flesh and bone of the body, then become dominant or prevailing. In summary Bailey states, ". . . the individual 'seeds' have portions of all things in fusion, but in each, some one thing prevails: the compound body is formed of seeds in juxtaposition, but in each body 'seeds' of one kind are in the majority with others latent among them themselves varying in number and kind."[33]

This is indeed an explanation of change on an atomistic basis, but it is a qualitative and not a quantitative atomism. With Anaxagoras it is no problem to derive the various qualities of things, because the qualities—whether of gold or flesh or bread—are primary *elements* which fuse, separate, and recombine. We might criticize the theory because the quantitative aspect is not adequately represented. Infinite divisibility, and the presence of everything in everything, are notions very divergent from the quantitative atomism that later became prevalent.

Very important in Anaxagoras' general theory is the concept of *Nous* or Mind. This was a principle of movement, a directing force responsible for the order that is manifest in the world. It is thus a "substance" analogous to the Love or Strife of Empedocles, and should be mentioned here for comparison with later atomism. *Nous,* said Anaxagoras, "is infinite and self-ruled, and is mixed with nothing, but is alone, itself by itself. . . . For it is the thinnest of all things and the purest, and has all knowledge about everything and . . . has power over all things . . . that have life."[34] It is the source of movement and life, the cause of things, and a teleological principle. *Nous* does not represent a personal deity or a theistic concept, but it does introduce a certain element of purpose and design into the world.

The history of ideas presents a vigorous drama of conflicting attitudes. When we try to explain the world, we must account for the various qualities and their changes that we perceive, but we must furnish an account that is intellectually satisfying. There are those philosophers who stress the qualitative aspects while others claim the primacy of quantitative factors. The foremost doctrine of this latter type is that of classical atomism, generally associated with Democritus (460–370 B.C.). The doctrine, originated probably by Leucippus and popularized by Lucretius, represents a tremendous achievement which grew naturally from the theories of the earlier Greeks. This new atomism was in essence strictly quantitative, while qualities were relegated to a secondary position. The ultimate or truly real elements were particles that were considered to be qualitatively the same. They were not air or earth or fire or water, or any material recognizable by the senses. The atoms could be appreciated only in thought. Their ultimate composition was not in any way a sensible property.

Atoms, however, were not entirely similar one to the other, since they differed in shape and size. Some were big; some were little. They had diverse shapes, with various humps, depressions, grooves, and hooks, which allowed the atoms to interlace and join together in various combinations. Furthermore, the atoms were constantly in motion. Thus, classical atomism maintained that there was one ultimate substance, divided into multiple simple irreducible particles of varying shape and size that were in constant movement, moving in empty space.

The world that we see and know arises from different combinations of these elements. The atoms differing in shape, size, weight, arrangement, and position, even though qualitatively alike, combine and recombine, and serve as building blocks for the individual objects. Change is the recombination of atoms. It is the atoms which are real and which constitute Existence.

But how do qualities arise out of atoms? This is a very difficult problem, for in classical atomism all the various qualities are secondary and derivative and, contrary to the teachings of Anaxagoras, have no independent reality. They arise only from the act of perception, that is, from the interaction, somehow, of soul-atoms and other atoms. What we call a quality is an interaction between soul-atoms and atoms of the thing perceived. The reality is the atomic structure. Qualities are not "really real." If this formulation does not appear satisfactory, we must realize that it inheres in every materialistic philosophy.

Materialistic doctrines based on atomism were very popular in certain medical circles but, as we shall see, Galen was bitterly opposed to all such interpretations. On the contrary, he was concerned particularly with qualities rather than with quantities, and drew his doctrines largely from Aristotle. For Aristotle change was very real, and qualities were very real, yet a quantitative view cannot be discarded. There resulted what we can only call a hybrid, that is, a combination of elemental qualities and elemental or simple bodies. For Aristotle the traditional earth, air, fire, and water were "apparently" simple bodies, but actually were "blended" out of qualities.[35] The four elemental qualities, the hot and the cold, the moist and the dry, exist not as isolated entities, but as pairs of opposites, each of which, it might be said, exerts a reciprocal tension on the other. Each of the simple bodies is characterized by a different pair of qualities. "For Fire is hot and dry, whereas Air is hot and moist . . . and Water is cold and moist, while Earth is cold and dry."[36] Contrary to Empedocles, who denied transformation of elements, Aristotle maintained that the elemental qualities could replace one another, and as the replacement occurred, the substance would also change. There would be a real transformation. Each element had a characterizing pair of qualities, one of which was shared with another element. Thus, "air" and "fire" both possessed the primary quality "hot," but differed in respect to the other member of the pair. A change in a single quality would also change the character of the element—if "dry" turned into "moist," then "fire" would change into "air." Similarly, if we regard the quotation above, we can see that "earth" can easily result from "water," and "fire" from "earth," since their characterizing qualities have a factor in common.[37] But to change "fire" into "water" would be more difficult, involving alteration in both members of the quality-pairs.

Aristotle's formulation stressed the reality of change. The concept of four primary qualities was very ancient—Hippocrates discussed the "hot" and the "cold" as abstract causative principles in disease—but Aristotle organized a coherent and influential doctrine, which, coupled with his own elaborate metaphysics, preserved aspects of both Empedocles and Anaxagoras (and Plato as well), and provided a rallying point for those who opposed the atomism of Democritus.

IV

Physiological activity depends on the basic qualities already discussed; for, said Galen, "Bodies act upon and are acted upon by each other in virtue of the Warm, Cold,

Moist and Dry. And if one is speaking of any activity, whether it be exercised by vein, liver, arteries, heart, alimentary canal, or any part, one will be inevitably compelled to acknowledge that this activity depends upon the way in which the four qualities are blended."[38] The organs as they function alter the various substances into qualities appropriate to the part involved.[39]

Even a casual glance at functions such as growth or nutrition indicates their complexity. It is very obvious that bone is different from kidney and both are different from brain, yet the same food will nourish all organs. To explain all this is a challenge which Galen met by a series of analyses, part of which we will try to follow.

Nutrition and growth are mediated by the blood, a common store from which the different organs selectively draw what is appropriate. The first major problem in analysis, then, is the transformation of food into blood. This takes place in stages, of which the first is the alteration of food into chyle. That is, the ingested food loses its original qualities and takes on certain new properties, intermediate to the formation of blood. Some digestive changes were recognized as taking place in the mouth,[40] but chylification occurs chiefly in the stomach. The transformation cannot take place at once, but requires several stages. After the chyle is formed, the nutritious substances must be absorbed, and the superfluous eliminated. Galen appreciated the "specialization" involved, and believed that separate functions required separate organs for accomplishment. Hence the multiplicity of bodily organs, all concerned with nutrition.

The production of chyle in the stomach had long been familiar. To explain its formation Erasistratus had invoked a mechanical process. He claimed that the grinding power of the stomach contractions produced softening of the food and removal of waste.[41] But Galen, with keen perception, had no use for simple mechanical explanations. Digestion was not a process whereby foodstuffs broke down into smaller and smaller particles of the same character. Instead, there was a change which yielded not a smaller edition of the original, but quite a different substance. By analogy, a baker does not produce bread merely by grinding the constituents up fine. Instead, through a number of operations including moisture and heat and fermentation, bread will result. Digestion in the stomach was somewhat similar. It was a "coction," that is, a cooking, during which the food changed its quality.[42] Such coction and resulting change were part of chylification, which in turn was part of blood formation.

The alteration which digestion produced depended on the innate heat. This, centering in the heart, we can regard as the ancient equivalent of metabolism. The stomach was in a specially favorable position to alter the ingesta, since the surrounding viscera—liver and spleen to the sides, heart above, and the omentum sheltering them all (see p. 48)—concentrated the heat, "like a lot of burning hearths around a great cauldron."[43]

The food, "subdued" and "altered"[44] in the stomach, passed into the intestines whose primary function was to distribute the nutrient material into the absorbing veins. However, the intestines also had a secondary function of further elaborating the nutrient.[45] The superfluities, which were not absorbed, were excreted. In the course of his detailed analysis Galen made many trenchant physiological observations. He knew the action of the pyloric sphincter and appreciated many data regarding gastric retention and the digestive and absorptive functions in the small intestine.[46]

Transformation of chyle into blood began in the absorbing (or portal) veins which went from the intestine to the liver, but the liver was the primary organ of blood formation. Galen had a sound appreciation of liver structure, recognizing different components, such as veins, arteries, nerves, bile passages, covering membranes, and the parenchyma or "flesh." Each component had its function.[47] All tended to blood formation but the parenchyma of the liver was the major site of sanguification, the others, subsidiary. Galen, who tried to infer function from structure, frequently made shrewd observations and guesses about the different digestive organs.

The foregoing paragraphs indicate very sketchily what Galen called "alteration," or the transformation of one substance into another quite different. He enumerated and described the various steps that comprised the function of digestion. He accounted for the function by boldly proclaiming a "faculty of alteration" which existed in the body. It is, of course, perfectly true that "explaining" an activity as a "faculty" adds no new knowledge. To say that something happens because there is a power which makes it happen, seems to be on a par with asking a small child why he did thus-and-so, and receiving the reply, "Because I wanted to." We have not made any progress. Nevertheless, Galenic "faculties," beaten almost to death by wits, logicians, historians, and scientists, should not be dismissed as merely a source of merriment. The concept focuses attention on biology as a separate discipline, with its own characteristic problems. The "faculties" emphasize that biology is dynamic; that vital phenomena, involving real change and temporal sequence, can be studied as functional units; that description and analysis represent the first stage of understanding. And as we shall see, the "faculties" indicate that shallow explanations must be avoided; that the scientist may probe for biological and physical similarities among phenomena; that a broad synoptic viewpoint may be of value, even though specific details may be incorrect. These implications should not be lightly disregarded.

Galen showed that the "faculty of alteration" depended on certain definite anatomical structures and had certain definite functional correlates with normal and abnormal states. Some of the normals we have already indicated. In many disease states, such as fevers or disturbance of innate heat, the digestion would be impaired. In describing such facts Galen was recording and tying together various observed sequences, correlating them with other observations and with inferences (some of which were sound, others not). Galen was putting "envelopes" around clusters of facts. Out of the entire flux of events he selected some as going together, as possessing some inner unity and coherence. These he isolated in an individual envelope, and each envelope he called a separate faculty. The name added nothing. The significant feature was the description, analysis, and correlation, the perception that certain biologic features belong together, and are separable from others. "Faculty" we can construe as a shorthand way of recording, describing, and analyzing data. There were many different faculties, which means that facts and sequences can be analyzed in many different modalities.

It is important to grasp the scope of Galen's concepts, clothed as they are in the language of faculties. "Alteration" is merely one among many, and is only an early stage in the total process of nutrition. The ingested food, after many transformations, must eventually be utilized by separate tissues. The formation of blood, and its distribution throughout the body, are not enough. For every tissue there must be a *presentation,* an *adhesion,* and an *assimilation.*

Galen's archaic terminology still has a surprisingly modern significance. Let us clarify his meaning with a few examples. Imagine a patient with arteriosclerosis, whose coronary arteries are very narrow. We might say that he has "coronary insufficiency," that is, although there is plenty of blood in the body, the narrow coronary arteries cannot furnish enough blood to satisfy the needs of the heart. Galen would say that there is a defective faculty of presentation, another way of saying that the heart does not get enough blood.

Or, in certain types of edema, the excess fluid readily runs off when the waterlogged tissues are punctured. We would say that the extra-cellular spaces are loaded with fluid, but Galen called this a defect in the *adhesive* faculty. That is, the fluid is "presented" but does not "stick." On the other hand, in certain types of inflammatory edema, an incision does not yield much fluid, even though the part is obviously swollen. We might explain this in terms of hydrophil proteins, osmotic pressures, and lymphatic blockage. But Galen noted the facts and referred to them as failure of *assimilation*. That is, the fluid was *presented* and *adhered,* but it did not become assimilated into the tissue.[48] Or, a diabetic may have a very high blood sugar. The blood vessels bring to the liver abundant glucose which that organ cannot utilize. We say that there is an insulin deficiency. Galen would have blamed a defective assimilative faculty.

Before we assess further the concept of faculties, let us examine some other modalities. Certain organs exert a *retentive* faculty. The uterus, for example, retains the embryo until the gestation period is complete. At term the mouth of the womb opens and the eliminative faculty, previously dormant, takes over to expel the fetus.[49] The same faculty controls other organs. The stomach, the gall bladder, the urinary bladder, the rectum, all retain their appropriate contents, until a certain point at which the eliminative faculty takes over.[50]

Now Galen has here performed two distinct services. In

the first place, he had described the activity of certain hollow organs. Description of natural phenomena is the first step in science. The scientist must be able to observe accurately and describe clearly. But Galen has taken a further and very significant step. By invoking a common "faculty" applicable to several different organs, he has in effect declared a relationship between them. The discharge of bile, urine, feces, products of conception—each represents a single example of expulsion. Galen perceived a common thread between these various phenomena. He did not know anything about smooth muscle, autonomic nervous system, circulating hormones, or other paraphernalia of modern physiology, applicable to these organs. But despite his ignorance Galen did homologize diverse phenomena. The "expulsive faculty" represents a generalization that various bodily activities, in widely different modalities, all had something in common. "Faculty" indicates the unity, but does not analyze any further than to say that these observed phenomena are related. Later research discovered the existence of smooth muscle and defined the relationship more closely. Yet the original perception, that a functional relationship exists, is a far from negligible attainment.

The scientist is one who can perceive a common thread of relation among diverse phenomena. The terminology is less important than the flash of recognition which somehow glimpses the universal within the many particulars. To be sure, this interest in homologizing various functions and perceiving inner connections among things has often led to serious error. But it is nevertheless part of that essential scientific attitude, which constantly seeks deeper and broader interconnections among phenomena. This search—call it research if you will—is sometimes successful, sometimes not.

Extremely important was the faculty of "attraction"

which existed in many different modalities, and whose examination is quite instructive in understanding Galen's thinking. As already emphasized, the blood furnishes to the different organs all the materials necessary for nutrition and growth. How does it happen that the heart-nutriment goes specifically to the heart and nowhere else, and that the bones receive exactly what they need, and not something foreign? In other words, how can we account for *specificity,* of which there are so many exquisite examples? In a sense the history of physiology represents the progressive clarification of this single problem. Galen had his own answer, which centered on the concept of specific attraction.

He noted two kinds of attraction. One type is exemplified by the filling of a vacuum: when a bellows expands, air rushes in. This really is a mechanical property and is of a rather different order from the second type, which is truly specific[51] and therefore depends on special and peculiarly appropriate relationships. An example of the latter is the attraction between iron and a magnet, or between amber and chaff. Certain facts of magnetism and static electricity had long been recognized but there remained the problem of connecting them with other phenomena. Galen's general method was to show that all other explanations offered were unsatisfactory, so that invoking a "faculty" was all that was left. He realized quite clearly— at least in some passages—that "faculty" was a stopgap, designed to eliminate unsatisfactory explanations, and explicitly declared, "So long as we are ignorant of the true essence of the cause which is operating, we call it a *faculty.* Thus we say there exists in the veins a blood-making faculty . . . and in each of the other parts a special faculty corresponding to the function or activity of that part."[52] To study the faculties it was important to study the effects (i.e., the observed phenomena), from which we can work backward to the cause.

Now, regarding the observed facts of magnetism, the Epicurean or atomistic explanation was that certain atoms flow from the lodestone, others from the iron. These atoms have similarities in shape, and hence can become entangled and interlocked one with the other. This Galen considered to be nonsense, "For, that these small corpuscles belonging to the lodestone rebound, and become entangled with other similar particles of the iron, and that by means of this entanglement (which cannot be seen anywhere) such a heavy substance as iron is attracted—I fail to understand how anybody could believe this." Ought we to believe, "That, forsooth, some of the particles that flow from the lodestone collide with the iron and then rebound back, and that it is by these that the iron becomes suspended?"[53] Obviously, the answer is no.

Galen presented many observations regarding magnetic phenomena which rendered such an explanation quite unacceptable. In this, of course, he was exhibiting the most approved scientific method, namely, drawing the logical implications of a theory, then studying the observed facts, finding that these facts were not consistent with the theoretical demands, and indicating that the theory was therefore untenable. Unfortunately, this he did chiefly in controversy when trying to disprove someone else's theory. He was not ordinarily so sound when trying to demonstrate his own position in a positive fashion. Galen's own "explanation" was that there existed a specific attractive faculty, operative between the lodestone and the iron. This has at least two merits. It refuses to accept a manifestly inadequate hypothesis; and it indicates a peculiarly circumscribed set of phenomena, apparently *sui generis,* with highly specific properties.

Actually Galen pointed to numerous different areas,

each quite circumscribed and limited, and each showing a *specific* relationship among particular objects or processes. An amusing example concerns hygroscopic action. He described what was apparently a well-known trick among farmers who, bringing corn to the city, want to steal some without being detected. They "fill earthen jars with water and stand them among the corn; the corn then draws the moisture into itself through the jar and acquires additional bulk and weight."[54] Yet, Galen pointed out, if you place the same vessel in the very hot sun, there is very little water loss. The conclusion is, that corn has a specific power of drawing to itself moisture which is in its neighborhood. We, who eschew faculties, prefer to speak of hygroscopic action. Galen was ignorant of this concept, but he did indicate that water loss through evaporation could be vastly less than the loss to a hygroscopic agent, and indicated further a specificity to this behavior.

Specific action is especially important in biology. Drugs, for example, may be highly specific, a fact already well known to Hippocrates. A particular drug would draw off, or attract, a particular humor. Furthermore, Galen believed that certain drugs were highly specific against certain poisons, or against foreign bodies. These phenomena he explained by specific attraction—"that everything which exists possesses a faculty by which it attracts its proper quality, and that some things do this more, and some less."[55] It is scarcely necessary to point to the present-day antibiotics and other specific drugs. But we might mention that when research organizations systematically test thousands of compounds, searching for specific antibacterial or anticancer potency, they are implicitly accepting Galen's belief, expressed above.

Galen's analysis of kidney function illustrates the attractive faculty especially clearly. He assumed, to start with, that urine existed as waste matter in the blood.

The problem was to determine how it became separated from the blood. Galen demonstrated quite clearly that the kidneys served this separatory function. One possibility, that "the urine is conveyed by its own power to the kidneys,"[56] he did not take seriously and dismissed without further ado. This left two possibilities: either the blood vessels propel the blood into the kidneys, or the kidneys attract the urine from the blood. He showed to his own satisfaction that there was no propulsive action. Hence the only remaining possibility was an attractive faculty.[57]

We must realize that Galen's modes of investigation were quite limited. Although he practiced vivisection and drew many important conclusions therefrom, he obviously could not perform microdissection, or study capillary filtration, membrane equilibrium, blood and urine chemistry, and selective reabsorption. Since he had to draw the best conclusions he could from the data that he did possess, he relied somewhat more on argument than we would today.

His arguments are interlocking and actually involve a serious begging of the question. Thus, if the veins (or in modern terms, the blood vessels) did exert a propulsive action, there would be two necessary conditions: the kidneys would have to act like sieves or filters; and all the blood in the body would have to pass through those filters. Unless these requirements were fulfilled, the hypothesis would be logically untenable. But in regard to the blood such a sieve-like action could not take place, for "if the blood were destined to be purified by them [i.e., the kidneys] as if they were sieves, the whole of it [the blood] would have to fall into them, the thin part being thereafter conveyed downwards, and the thick part retained above."[58] But this is impossible, since the kidneys lie not in the direct course of these vessels but are situated on each side. How could blood get to these organs? Only through the renal vessels (the veins, as he thought). If the kidneys actually performed a filtration, Galen admitted that the blood within the renal veins might be so purified, and the urine contained therein might be removed by filtration. But then the purified residue within the renal vessels would obstruct any new blood from finding its way in. How could purified blood be removed from the renal veins to allow new blood to enter?[59]

The circularity of the reasoning is apparent. For filtration to take place the vessels must propel the blood to the kidney. For this to be effective there would have to be a propulsion of *all* the blood in the body, that is, a circulation. But all the blood does not get propelled. How did he know? Because there is no circulation. Hence all the blood does not pass through the kidneys. The entire argument rests on the basic premise, accepted without proof, that the blood does not circulate. Therefore there was no way in which all the blood could pass through the kidneys, and so, even if the kidneys were sieves, all the blood could not be filtered through them. Since by this reasoning the kidneys do not act as sieves, then the only way in which they could remove the urine from the blood was to exert "traction," that is, an attractive faculty.

It is interesting to imagine what would have happened had Galen adopted a different premise. Supposing he had assumed, even without proof, that the kidneys *did* act as sieves or filters. Then, in order for this to take place, he would have had to make the logical assumption that the blood *did* circulate. He would have arrived at this conclusion by pure reason. Having achieved this proposition as a postulate, he might have been led to investigate the matter experimentally. Everything depends on the initial premises, which are accepted without proof.

The faculty of attraction had certain merits. Like the other faculties, it directed attention to particular sequences. It homologized the action of various body components. We today know a great deal about cells, how they work and how they react, how they absorb and utilize nutritive substances. Galen did not know any of these data, did not know the units we call cells. But he did appreciate that widely different organs exerted certain functions in common, that these functions were complex, and that one aspect thereof could be designated "attraction." With all this we cannot quarrel.

Through his faculty of attraction Galen went too far afield. He tried to homologize activities that to our eyes cannot be closely related. Hygroscopic action on the one hand and excretion of urine on the other, each involve phenomena with specific properties in a distinctive pattern. But just because each activity presented its own pattern does not mean that the patterns themselves were related. We cannot see a significant relation between all the different activities which he labeled "attraction." Magnetism and specific drug action and kidney excretion do not appear to have any over-all unity. We must say that Galen is wrong. But we will not say that he is "foolish."

A faculty, as Galen used the term, represents to our modern sense a unit of description, and not in any sense an explanation. Phenomena fall into recurrent patterns which are predictable. "Faculty" is a shorthand way of saying: such a sequence exists, even though we cannot indicate its mechanisms; these sequences are not only regular but exhibit a sort of unity in time, with a beginning, a middle, and an end; when we are at the beginning, we know what is going to come; when we are at the end, we know what has preceded. We might offer an analogy, and compare a Galenic faculty to a phonograph record. If we want to use Galenic and Aristotelian terms, we can say that the record is the potentiality of a performance which can become an actuality when we place it on the machine.

77

When the record is being played, we have an active functioning (*energeia*); when it is finished, we have a completed activity (*ergon*). At any moment while it is being played, there is still an undisclosed potentiality (*dynamis*) in the process of becoming actual. The phonograph record which we hold in our hand we can call not only the potentiality of a performance, but in a sense its *cause*.[60] The record represents a unified whole, has the power, so to speak, of producing the effect, and is analogous to the "faculty."

In biology we have emphasized the important difference between describing phenomena and explaining them. Our analogy indicates a similar difference between listening to the music and explaining how it came about. Once we have the record we can reproduce the music as often as we want and can become extremely familiar with every nuance. But there is a vast difference between being thus familiar and understanding the responsible mechanisms. These are separable into two areas. One concerns the technique of recording and reproduction and embraces the sciences of acoustics and electronics, as well as the chemistry of plastics and related subjects. Any of these subjects might require a lifetime's study to master the details fully. On the other hand there is a totally different area concerned with the psychological and cultural factors which produced the music. If we want to understand or "explain" a late Beethoven quartet that we hear on a record, the techniques that made possible the recording or reproduction are only one aspect. We must also consider the personality of Beethoven. How can we analyze his genius? In what relation did he stand to his era? How did he transform music? What was his influence? The rather barbarous term "musicology" can be used to embrace the relation to his music of psychology, history, sociology, and aesthetics—again a field which could absorb a lifetime.

But fortunately, to hear the quartet, and to enjoy it, we do not need all this knowledge. The record by itself is a self-contained whole for certain purposes. The record comprises a sequence of phenomena exhibiting inner connections which can also integrate with other comparable sequences. The "explanations" for the record and its music are indeed important but *for most purposes* they are not necessary. Certainly, millions who listen to records have only the slightest knowledge of all the "explanatory" background material.

We suggest that the difference between playing a record and knowing how the music came into being is comparable to the difference between description and explanation. The Galenic faculties are like phonograph records. They are bundles which describe various physiological processes. These bundles, like records, can be compared and arranged. They can be replaced by newer and improved versions. They can be very useful in many practical affairs. But they do not of themselves furnish any explanation of how they came to be. To achieve such an explanation we must go beyond the record itself and must deal with other factors.

There are many practical situations where explanations are not particularly important, where we want to know *what* will happen rather than *why* it will happen. Description alone can be entirely satisfactory in such circumstances. Galen's great contributions were in describing various factual sequences and transformations, and perceiving similarities among natural phenomena. His observations were those we call "natural history." Despite what he often said, he stressed observation rather than explanation. The faculties, when understood in this light, should not be objects of scorn.

79

V

Galen was very valiant in refuting hypotheses he did not like, and often revealed great experimental skill and keen reasoning to make his point. For example, he demonstrated very conclusively that the bladder urine came from the kidneys via the ureters, and not, as Asclepiades claimed, through a condensation of vapors.[61] His experiments and reasoning are models of sound method.

He insisted that we must bow before facts, although sometimes this humility was deceptive. Like most of us, Galen had the greatest respect for facts when they fitted in with his own ideas, but he tended to ignore those which were not so accommodating. Yet Galen knew perfectly well the potency of brute fact. He expressed himself so clearly that modern writers on scientific method can scarcely improve his statements. Speaking of proper education he declared that the young man should have a most ardent love of truth, and devote himself day and night, "to learn thoroughly all that has been said by the most illustrious of the Ancients. And when he has learnt this, then for a prolonged period he must test and prove it, observing what part of it is in agreement, and what in disagreement with obvious fact; then he will choose this and turn away from that."[62] Again, in one of his controversies, he severely criticized Asclepiades for pursuing hypotheses which ran counter to observation. "Much better would it have been for him not to assail obvious facts, but rather to devote himself entirely to these."[63]

This leads to a methodological problem of extreme importance, the relationship of what we actually observe to what we infer. We have seen how Hippocrates depended on the eye of reason to penetrate beyond the manifest appearances. "Reason" may be more important than observation. We can, for example, point to the sleight-of-hand artist, who shows us extraordinary phenomena which we label "illusions." We call them illusions because the "eye of reason" tells us they must be. When we see a torn piece of paper rendered whole again, we say it didn't "really" happen. We mistrust our senses in favor of our intellectual construct. What, then, will we say, when Galen pokes fun at Asclepiades, alleging that he disregarded the evidence of his senses and accepted instead what his reason indicated must be the truth?[64]

Unfortunately, Galen had a double standard regarding the "eye of reason." It was very praiseworthy when he employed it, but when his opponents attempted its exercise, there resulted only rash and unfounded hypotheses. The history of thought repeatedly illustrates this dichotomy—my reasoning leads to truth, but you, who reason improperly, can achieve only error. The eighteenth century was much concerned with hypothesis and the "justness" of reasoning, continuing a tradition in which Galen took a prominent part. But this attitude is not restricted to any era or country. Instead, it is a major failing of the human mind to outrun the evidence, and to leap to conclusions which the facts will not support. Whoever makes this inductive leap believes he is adequately supported. But a changed perspective and new knowledge may indicate how wrong he actually was.

There is no perversity of spirit involved. Mankind must always think or act within a definite and limited framework. It is "natural" to seek explanations and to make inferences within the confines that are familiar and comfortable. One culture attributes disease quite "naturally" to spirits, while a different culture just as readily invokes bacteria or allergies. Galen was not at all unique. He could not transcend the framework within which he moved.

We must realize that we cannot completely separate "facts" from "theories," or "percept" from "concept."

Mental life is an indissoluble blend of concrete and abstract. This blend is the matrix of all thinking. What we call fact and theory, percept and concept, observation and inference, are separations that are very useful but nevertheless quite artificial. However much we claim to regard "facts," we are necessarily influenced by all those abstractions and conceptual attitudes that comprise our mental environment, which we can no more shed than we can shed our skin.

In this respect Galen was no exception. He did offer his own explanations, but in so doing, he too had a framework that limited and directed his thinking, a framework constructed of *qualities* and *humors*. Regarding these he simply did not have the objective or critical attitude that he maintained toward atomism. His statements, as we see them, go way beyond the evidence, exhibit confusion, and certainly lack precision. The four qualities, for example, were sometimes regarded as sensory qualities, at other times as metaphysical properties. Yet Galen did not keep these usages separate.

We are quite accustomed to the multiple and quite distinct meanings that a single word may display. The single term "dry," for example, may refer to many different objects, and have a different sense for each. Dry sand is in a very different category from dry wine, and both are distinct from dry wit. Ordinarily we avoid confusion without difficulty. But Galen often faltered and confused his meanings. For example, the concept "hot" referred sometimes to a property resident in objects as a sensible caloric quality; sometimes to a substance which could produce heat at a future time (that is, something potentially hot); other times to the innate heat in living bodies. The term "dry" meant sometimes that sensory quality which was opposite to moist; at other times it was the effect produced, rather than the quality. When Galen wanted to draw inferences or prove a point, he would casually shift meanings. Evidence intended for one meaning he would apply to a totally different meaning where that evidence might be quite irrelevant.

Galen wanted to correlate the four qualities with the four humors. The blood, we have seen, derives from the food. The transformation takes place in the absorbing veins and in the liver. But how do the other humors arise? For his answer Galen relied on the old concept of right measure or proportion, and the traditional four qualities. When the nutriment is absorbed into the veins, and subjected to the innate heat, blood is produced when that heat has the appropriate moderation. Otherwise, when the heat is not in the proper proportion, the other humors are produced. But the character of the food also was significant, for those foods "which are by nature warmer are more productive of bile, while those which are colder produce more phlegm."[65] And Galen also applied the term "hot" and "cold" to periods of life, occupations, seasons, and natures. When any of these were "warmer" there was a tendency to produce bile; when they were "colder," phlegm.

Confusion there obviously is. We can appreciate how some of it arose, when Galen attended to similarities which we would call superficial, and neglected differences which we regard as significant. Thus, mucus is relatively cold to the touch; coryza is more frequent in cold weather; old people who have "thin blood" feel chilly more readily than do younger persons; old people lack the emotions that characterize youth, and in addition are subject to certain diseases that usually do not affect younger individuals. All these statements are true. If we want, we can make them all revolve around the term "cold" and thus claim a relationship. Those ailments prevalent in winter it is perhaps not unreasonable to call "cold" diseases. It is rather more of a stretch, but still plausible, to call old age a "cold age" because elderly people have failing hormonal and circulatory responses. But it is too great a strain on the theory to call various degenerative and infectious diseases "cold" because they afflict the aged who previously have been labeled "cold." If we regard all these usages as equivalent, and use them interchangeably; if we disregard all the differences as non-existent or inconsequential, then we can "prove" a great deal. But the proof ceases to be convincing whenever we begin to appreciate the distinctions.

Yet this criticism is not entirely fair, because it is only retrospectively that we note the confusion. That is, only after a discrimination has been made by someone else, do we realize the former lack of precision. If we do not know why old people feel chilly when younger individuals are quite comfortable, we may accept the term "cold" as primary. When differences do not impress themselves upon us, it is pardonable to neglect them. The whole history of medicine is, perhaps, a progressive discrimination. Someone with special insight, or special technique, is able to point out a distinction that had previously gone unnoticed. What seemed simple is found to be complex: what seemed unitary is found to be multiple. But there is an opposite and compensatory trend, for as differences multiply, new relationships are noted which connect up the multiplicity. The process is unending, one into many, and the many back into one, but always, like an ascending spiral, reaching new levels.

All periods contribute new discriminations and new relationships, but sometimes we can note a strong forward surge, at other times a slow consolidation. The great periods of advance are those which enlarge the framework that limits man's thinking; permit him to question concepts that he held uncritically; introduce new concepts, create new categories, and thus allow a re-evaluation of old data. Once we start to re-evaluate old ideas, we may break through our preconceptions. Such an expansion necessarily comes gradually, for many hard-working individuals must first chip away at the bonds. When we regard intellectual history in this light, we find that Galen was a systematizer who consolidated knowledge within an established framework, rather than a pioneer toward a new horizon.

The Philosophic Approach

PARACELSUS

Paracelsus (1493–1541) was a stormy and controversial figure during his life and has remained so through the centuries that followed. Philippus Aureolus Theophrastus Bombastus Paracelsus von Hohenheim, to give his full name, was born in Einsiedeln, Switzerland, the son of a physician. Very little is known about his early life. Van Helmont[1] declared that he had been castrated by a sow. Although this cannot be accepted as established historical fact, nevertheless his behavior and manner, the tone of his writings, his boasting and quarrelsome disposition, his incessant travel and inability to adapt for any length of time to any one place, all suggest some type of severe personality defect. His education was rather spotty, its extent obscure. There is no sound evidence that he ever secured a medical degree, but he did practice medicine and surgery, in itinerant fashion. Indeed, his life was that of a wanderer, constantly rebelling against authority, making a few friends and disciples, but very many enemies, and always finding it expedient not to stay very long in any one place. He attacked traditional theories and practice, antagonized all academic or professional authority, yet he courted popularity while achieving only a small nucleus of followers.

A tremendous critical literature has arisen regarding Paracelsus, his relation to his time, his writings, and his influences. In general, readers may find any desired shade of critical opinion. The extremes appear especially prominent. For example, in the seventeenth century, Francis Bacon declared of him that he "deserves to be separately chastised as a Monster . . . [for] like a sacrilegious Imposter, he has mixed and polluted divine Things with natural, sacred with profane, Fables with Heresies . . . [and] he has . . . magnified the absurd Pretences of Magicians, countenanced such Extravagances . . . being at once the Work and Servant of Imposture." And as for his followers, "By wandering through the Wilds of Experience they sometimes stumble upon useful discoveries; not by reason but by accident, whence proceeding to form theories, they plainly carry the Smoak and Tarnish of their art along with them. . . ."[2] Temkin quoted an eighteenth-century critic, that Paracelsus "lived like a pig, looked like a coachman and took most pleasure in the company of the loosest and lowest mob," while "all his writings seem to have been written during intoxication."[3] And the nineteenth-century historian Daremberg referred to various Paracelsian writings as "extravagant," "fantastic," the "hallucinations of a disordered mind," as "verbiage" or a "galimatias," as "virtually without meaning."[4]

On the other hand, there are those who praise him highly. One modern scholar declared in measured periods:

What makes this man great as thinker and physician is the anti-intellectualism of his attitude, his fearlessness with which he smashed icons of the ancients, particularly Galen . . . the vigor with which he extolled the ethical calling of the physician, the clarity with which he perceived the huge pattern on which both God and the physician weave and nature provides the loom and all the essentials. He became a martyr of natural science because he rejected speculation in favor of experience; a martyr of religion, for he built his theology without the church on a harmonious operation of God, nature, and man; a martyr of the good life, for he was searching for the basis of medical practice in love. . . .[5]

We find it quite impossible to accept this latter evaluation, but the earlier diatribes are equally one-sided. Most modern scholars achieve a balanced view, neither ignoring obvious defects nor denying great achievements. Certainly the study of Paracelsus entails difficulty. Obscurities abound, the literal and figurative are intermingled, meanings lie hidden and contradictions are many. Yet even the intrinsic obscurities become somewhat less opaque if we can reconstruct the intellectual framework within which he moved. Daremberg, for example, great scholar that he was, lacked a sympathetic appreciation of the contemporary problems, lacked, we might say, a historical perspective. With appropriate perspective the problems and their solutions blend into a wider context, in which, to be sure, we may have obscurity but not absurdity, and certainly not a galimatias.

The philosophy of Paracelsus exhibits a prevailing character: it is *dynamic*. Activity is the very essence. More im-

88

portant than structure is function, which is carried on by various powers, forces, spirits, virtues, influences, and sympathies. These all occupy the center of the stage. They are at *work*. The universe is a seething mass of activity, most of which is hidden, completely invisible; while what lies on the surface and what the senses can readily perceive are not very important. Paracelsus wanted always to get beneath the surface, to study the secret powers and forces, to find the deeper connections and relations among things. But, if he wanted to go below the surface, just where could he go?

Today, when we want to penetrate beneath surface appearances, when we want to study the profound activity at work around us, we invoke bacteria and viruses, enzymes and hormones, molecules, atoms, and subatomic particles. These we believe to be the stuff that makes up our world. Obviously Paracelsus knew nothing of these, so he used terms derived from *his* intellectual environment.

Textbooks call Paracelsus a Renaissance figure, as if this tag automatically identified his place in history. But such a label tends to blur rather than clarify the complexity of the fifteenth and sixteenth centuries. We may very properly ask, When was the Renaissance? In some circles it was considered to begin with the fall of Constantinople. This provided a very exact reference point: before May 29, 1453, we had the Middle Ages, and after that date, the Renaissance. But even in a less exaggerated form, this definition is no longer acceptable. The contrast between the Renaissance and the preceding era no longer appears so sharp as it once was thought to be.[6] The more we regard any single aspect, the more we appreciate that alterations were never quite so sharp or so independent as they may appear at first glance. Collapse is not truly sudden, but is preceded by a long slow period of decay. And new developments, new trends and ideas, do not appear suddenly but have a slow gestation.

Paracelsus was indeed a rebel, who assailed and condemned the medical practitioners of his day and tried to renovate medical practice. But his rebellion was part of a wider movement, with many conflicting currents, and many deep roots. During this period the changes in medicine and related subjects were slower than in many other modalities and entailed many complex relationships.

The rise of humanism, for example, is peculiarly interesting to the medical historian. The fifteenth century witnessed the declining vitality of scholasticism. The traditional philosophy which had reached its peak with Thomas Aquinas became less and less responsive to changing attitudes, turned arid and pedantic and out of touch with the popular needs and aspirations; in brief, it grew old and querulous. Many other institutions, religious and political, were also decaying, although this was noteworthy more in retrospect than to the contemporary eye. Coincidentally there were many activities that exhibited a youthful upswing; of these the renewed interest in the classics has acquired especial importance, capturing the popular imagination perhaps to an undue degree. The revival of both Latin and Greek texts, the growth of textual criticism, renewed interest in the scriptures, the purification of Latin style, new translations of the classics, sympathy with the pagan spirit and the individual, all these were very important and influential, and helped form the humanist tradition. But only recently have historians stressed the antiscientific bias of the humanists.[7]

In the later Middle Ages, while speculative philosophy was exhibiting hardening of the arteries, progress in mathematics, physics, and mechanics as well as in the mechanical arts was considerable.[8] There was a strong development of science during the latter Middle Ages, but the humanists who scorned the scholastic tradition scorned equally the slow patient progress of science and technology that is only now achieving appreciation. And the humanist influence has so occupied the center of the stage that other trends have been relatively neglected.

Paracelsus, while not at all a humanist, did as a rebel share their disdain for scholasticism. But even though he turned his back on that particular branch of philosophy he, unlike the humanists, formed part of another movement which embraced alchemy in the wider sense.

We cannot understand Paracelsus without some insight into magic, alchemy, and astrology. The practitioners and theorists in these subjects exhibited two distinct trends: there was an orientation toward spiritual, "idealistic," and immaterial entities, which we might lump together as the "heavens" and which represented the abstract and speculative aspects. There was also a tendency toward concrete and very mundane affairs—the "earth," which represented the more practical and empirical. But while these two attitudes were originally united, they speedily diverged. Excessive concern with spirits led eventually to the excesses of mysticism and spiritualism, demonology and witchcraft, and a general "soft-headed" attitude; while mundane concerns, empirically based, led to more concrete achievements and, eventually, after many false turnings, to modern medical science. Paracelsus followed both of these trends which, during his life, were not clearly separable. Alchemy and astrology had a broad theoretical base, as well as practical and manipulative components. That these became quite influential in medicine was due largely to Paracelsus.

The humanists did not have an enduring program. Their exaggerated faith in ancient classical writers, as if "mere re-translation and textual criticism of ancient Greek writers" might improve medical science and practice,[9] proved unfounded. Disillusionment with the humanistic approach soon set in. When it became apparent that return to the classics would not solve any pressing medical problem, the doctrines of Paracelsus, with their emphasis on alchemy, began to make a greater appeal. During his life very few of his writings were published, but after his death his works aroused more interest and were extensively published. They helped to swell that enthusiasm for magic and alchemy that marked the later sixteenth and much of the seventeenth century.

Yet we must realize that Paracelsus himself developed out of a long tradition which extended back to early Greek philosophy, and which gradually became transformed during the late classical period and the entire Middle Ages. Only by tracing these roots can we appreciate what he represented and what he tried to achieve.

II

To understand Paracelsus we must achieve some measure of enthusiasm for certain philosophic problems which have had a long and influential history and which formed the general background of his thinking. We might center the discussion around the question, What is the source of movement and activity? This has always been a puzzle, and has traditionally been associated with the questions, What is the most real? or, What has the greatest value? Although these formulations sound obscure, they embody concepts that are generally familiar.

According to one formulation, the actual material which constitutes the world is intrinsically inert, while all motion or activating force proceeds from some other source which is separate from matter. This is most apparent in the distinction between body and soul. The body, by itself, is inert; the soul, which provides all movement and activity, is distinct from the body and comes from a different realm. When the soul is joined to a body, the latter is activated; when the soul departs from the body, all activity correspondingly departs and the body relapses into its state of inert matter. The soul has higher value than the body. The realm of souls has higher value and greater reality than the realm of matter. Other philosophic systems invoked other motive principles such as the *Love* and *Hate* of Empedocles; or the *Mind* of Anaxagoras. But in all these formulations *there is a distinct separation between that which moves or activates and that which is moved.* The active force, however formulated, has a higher value than that on which it acts, and, in many philosophic systems, a greater degree of reality.

There is, however, a contrary viewpoint, which holds that activity or motion is a property of matter, intrinsic and inseparable therefrom. In classical atomic theory, for example, the atoms, in ceaseless movement, combine and recombine, and there is no power or agency apart from the atoms. Even the "soul" was material. This means that some atoms were more subtle than others, and by virtue of their fineness they could act in the way we associate with living things. But, however fine, they were still atoms, and soul had no existence outside the world of matter.

The distinction between these two schools of thought is very important. If, as earlier thinkers believed, life is the capacity for self-movement, then either this power is intrinsic in material objects (a view which may be designated as materialism), or else the power of movement derives from a supra-sensible, more real world, distinct from the world of inert objects. This view we may call dualism (although there may be some technical objections to this usage).

Soul, then, may be the principle of activity which acts upon matter. But "matter" is a concept quite variable in its

93

meaning. We can think of it in a relatively crude sense, something like lumps of metaphysical plasticene, which the celestial machinery squeezes and molds into determinate shapes; or with a more subtle and delicate signification, as something indeterminate, the substrate of qualities, the "receptacle" of forms, the principle of potentiality, or sometimes as "not-being." Or, in an ethical sense, something responsible for what is evil or undesirable. Detailed analysis would carry us too far into metaphysics.

The Platonic tradition introduced the so-called *Ideas,* those eternal qualities, essences, properties, patterns, or forms, whose interpretation continues to engage the philosophic mind. The eternal ideas represent the perfect, universal, and changeless. They have true reality and value, and contrast with the mutable objects of our ordinary sensible world. The souls participated in this divine world of greater reality and value. This Platonic distinction between the divine and the material world is basic to the understanding of Paracelsus.

A further aspect derives especially from Aristotle. While the philosophy of Aristotle differs from that of Plato, just how great is the difference is a matter of dispute. There are those who tend to stress the differences and make a sharp contrast between the two philosophers; and there are others who minimize the differences and stress the similarities. We confess an inclination to the latter school. But while we may dispute the degree to which the Aristotelian teachings are implicit in Plato, Aristotle did exert his own very profound influence on later thought. In the present connection we would mention especially his concept of movement and activity, involving purpose or goal. Today purpose or final causes are "bad words," which might be scribbled on the walls of intellectual outhouses, but not used in polite scientific society. But an earlier tradition accepted Aristotle's concept of a goal serving as the *source* of movement by furnishing the terminus toward which an object strives. Quite familiar is the concept of God as the "unmoved mover," pure Form or Actuality, eternal and perfect, who, unmoved, is the source of all movement. The final cause is "the object of desire" which moves without being moved.[10] It is that "at which the action aims." It "produces motions by being loved"[11] and thus is the goal toward which all objects strive and thereby realize themselves.

As objects achieve a goal, they pass from the potential to the actual. Goal, striving, and activity, the transition from the potential or unrealized to the actual or realized, thus lie at the heart of things. The concept of purpose or striving grates on the hypersensitive modern ear and has been an important factor in the superficial modern discrediting of Aristotle. But whether we accept or reject this teleology, we must recognize its importance in the history of thought. Paracelsus made full use of the concept of goal, of an aspect implicit or potential within a thing, which would unroll or realize itself as the potentiality became actual. All of this is essentially Aristotelian.

A third very influential component of Paracelsus' thinking derived from the Stoic philosophy which was materialistic, but in a very special sense. For the Stoics everything is matter, which meant to them not something inert but something intrinsically dynamic. Activity permeates it at all points. This activity, however, is neither blind nor determined by chance, as with the atomists, but represents a divine and rational principle—i.e., God, the active rational principle and source of life, who is everywhere and pervades everything. This is what is meant by pantheism. Matter is alive, since it exhibits activity which is vital and divine, yet only matter exists. The whole material universe *is* a living being, of which God is the soul. But the soul is still material, that is, extremely fine and active matter, exhibiting purpose and goal. The individual person is a microcosm whose soul and body bear the same relation to each other as God and the world.

Another aspect of the Stoic philosophy, particularly stressed by Pagel,[12] is the *logoi spermatikoi*. This is variously translated as the rational seeds or germs of things, or seminal intelligences. They represent forces which are finely material, and which determine the specificity, course, and activity of objects. The *logoi* are dynamic factors derived from God to explain *process*. But since the *logoi* are material, we mention them here, as part of the materialistic doctrines which merged with the Platonic and Aristotelian tradition in Renaissance philosophy.

Platonism exerted its influence chiefly through the writings of Plotinus, which we must analyze in some detail. The chief problem was the relation of the perceptual world to the unseen world of higher reality. Plotinus (A.D. 204–70), who considered himself a follower of Plato and not an innovator, was very influential in shaping Christian doctrine, and also placed his imprint on medieval science and on Paracelsus.

Trying to explain the world, Plotinus began with the concept of God. What is the nature of God? How do we pass from God to the concrete world? For Plotinus, God was one, absolute, transcendent, beyond knowledge, beyond description; God was the Good, existing by and for himself. How, then, can we pass from such ineffable perfection to the concrete imperfect world around us? To solve the problem Plotinus had to postulate that the nature of perfection was to overflow and be fruitful.[13] Perfection must generate, must produce something other than itself, yet without detracting from or diminishing itself. The process of overflow, of generation-without-diminution, is called emanation. It takes place progressively and by necessity. There is not involved any fiat or act of will. It is simply the nature of perfection. Because God is perfect, emanations necessarily occur. Given this property, Plotinus could explain everything.

The first overflow or emanation results in an intellectual realm which is knowable and which corresponds roughly to the Platonic world of Ideas. It goes by a variety of terms, of which MacKenna prefers "Intellectual Principle." With this, the One has already become multiple, but the process does not thereby cease. "To this power [of emanation] we cannot impute any halt . . . [for] it must move forever outward, until the universe stands accomplished to the ultimate possibility. All, thus, is produced by an inexhaustible power giving its gift to the universe, no part of which it can endure to see without some share in its being."[14] All this, it must be emphasized, follows from the nature of Divinity.

Since the Intellectual Principle cannot rest, it in turn overflows to produce Soul, the second emanation. Soul is both one and many. There is the World-Soul, and also individual souls, and yet they are all one. Souls "are held together at the source much as light is a divided thing upon earth, shining in this house and that, and yet remains uninterruptedly one identical substance."[15] With Soul or souls, multiplicity becomes more pronounced.

God, Mind (or Intellectual Principle), and Soul constitute a trinity that is completely divine, yet exhibits a hierarchy. However, Plotinus still had to make the transition from the divine sphere to the mundane. Because the nature of Being is such that it must overflow in a descending chain, the material world is readily achieved. Said Plotinus, "In the absence of body, soul could not have gone forth, since there is no other place to which its nature would allow it to descend. Since go forth it must, it will generate a place for itself; at once body, also, exists."[16] At one stroke Plotinus bridged the gap between the divine or spiritual world, and the world of sense. Because there is the principle of emanation, the overflow of soul necessarily requires body. The one diffuses into many and the spiritual into the material.

The descent from soul to the concrete material world does not take place all at once. There is a graded hierarchy of souls. Those which remain closest to the All-soul have a minimum degree of corporality and, being closest to the Intellectual Principle, have the greatest intellectual aspect. But the further they descend from the All-soul, the greater the corporality. Celestial beings (that is, souls not embodied), man, animals, and plants, all have souls, but these differ one from the other and form an obvious hierarchy. They are at different loci in the process of emanation, and with progressively greater corporality they are progressively more distant from the intellectual world, or Intellectual Principle.[17]

Plotinus expressed what has been called the Principle of Plenitude, an idea which Lovejoy[18] has traced from Plato right up to modern times. The idea may be paraphrased, that the real, starting with God, manifests itself in a descending hierarchy of existence which cannot cease until every possible form has become manifest. There is, figuratively, a chain, reaching from the highest to the lowest, which embraces all possibilities. The higher examples have more of the divine essence, less of matter. As the divine component successively diminishes, the material component increases *pari passu*. But the unbroken sequence derives from God's nature which requires variety, expansion, and overflow.

Neo-Platonic doctrines were very influential in European thought, but their original form suffered various accretions and alterations which could be called degeneration. Especially important, with a long history of its own, is the Cabala, a strange blend that included among its components Neo-Platonic and Gnostic philosophy, Pythagorean number theory, and Jewish theosophy. The term Cabala or Kabbala originally signified doctrines received by tradition, but in the late Middle Ages came to indicate a fairly specific body of teachings which concerned the nature of God, the earth, intermediate beings, and man. The Cabala, like Neo-Platonism, relied on emanations in several series, which proceeded from God, like rays of light. These emanations bridged the gap between infinite and finite, and yielded progressive differentiation without in any way diminishing God's perfection. In the universe there were four different worlds, each of which was a decade of emanations, and each lower than its predecessor. Only in the fourth world, called "Asiah," with its ten emanations, do we encounter matter, that is, the world of change and corruption wherein dwell evil spirits, progressing downward to the Prince of Darkness.

The universe, however, was incomplete until man was created, man the microcosm, comprising and uniting in himself everything found in the great world above. Every part of man's being corresponds to some part of the visible universe. The comparison between man the microcosm, and the universe or macrocosm, dates back to early Greek philosophy. Heidel pointed out the basic root: to know what man is, we must know the nature of the world. Analogies between physics and biology indicate that "the laws of human physiology are in reality only special forms of universal laws."[19] Cabalistic doctrine can be construed as having its own "physics" and "physiology," although its vocabulary and concepts are very strange to present-day physicists or physiologists. We must realize, however, that the Cabala offered, in its way, a systematic description of the universe, a system within which any single event might find an explanation. The precise details are not relevant to our purpose. It is enough to appreciate that the

Cabala was one of the means by which Neo-Platonic thought was transmitted to the Renaissance.[20]

III

The concepts of magic, with their long and fascinating history,[21] were also vastly influential. There were certain impressive features. Magic was largely based on concrete experience, yet it depended on theory which was neither closely knit nor consistent. Magic was thus a composite of observations interpreted in the light of a particular philosophy. According to present-day standards the believers in magic seriously lacked sound critical or "scientific" judgment. A contemporary definition considered it to contain "the most profound contemplations of sacred things." But this was not all, for in addition it studied "the nature, power, quality, substance and vertues [*sic*]" of these things.[22] The "virtues" meant the peculiar properties and attributes—we might say "essences"—which inhere in some things but not in others.

One of the authors most influential in the sixteenth century was a slightly older contemporary of Paracelsus, Agrippa of Nettesheim (1486–1535), whose most significant work was written in 1510 when he was only twenty-four, but which was not published until 1531. It is the work of a young enthusiast, already very learned but not strikingly original. Most of the theoretical aspects may be found in earlier writers. Nevertheless, since his exposition is unusually clear, we may choose him to represent certain types of sixteenth-century magic.

Let us, then, look through his eyes and observe a few special "virtues" that exist in the world around us. An excellent example is the "power" of digestion. How does it happen that the food we eat undergoes such marked changes? Body or vital heat is one factor, but not the only

one. If heat were the only property involved, then, said
Agrippa, meat should be digested as well in front of the
fire as in the stomach. Since this obviously is not the case,
there must be, apart from the qualities which we know,
"other certain imbred [sic] vertues created by nature."[23]
Such a "virtue" is indeed something quite special, residing
specifically in the stomach, and not diffused throughout
nature.

Another splendid example of special power is the lodestone which attracts iron. There again is a very specific
phenomenon. Many stones may look very much alike, but
only one particular kind will show this power of attraction. There are many different metals but only one will be
attracted. Clearly there are some very special properties involved, not well understood but quite acceptably designated "virtue" or "power," quite distinct from the ordinary attributes of stones in general.

These two examples drawn from concrete experience
represent phenomena that are, and were, well recognized.
However, not all the examples are so well grounded in
experience. Agrippa boldly made many false assertions as
if they too had an equally sound empirical basis. Thus he
declared,

It is well known to all, that there is a Certain vertue in the
Loadstone, by which it attracts Iron, and that the Diamond
doth by its presence take away that vertue of the Loadstone:
so also Amber, and jeat rubbed, and warmed draw a straw to
them . . . [;] a Carbuncle shines in the dark, the stone aetites
put above the young fruit of Women, or Plants, strengthens
them, but being put under, causes abortion; the Jasper stench-
eth blood . . . [;] Rhubarb expels choller [sic]; the liver of
Camelion burnt, raiseth flowers, and thunders. The stone Helatropium dazles [sic] the sight, and makes him that wears it
to be invisible.[24]

All these statements were accepted as fact, and "well known" at that. Clearly there was a high index of credulity. Many so-called facts were accepted on rather tenuous evidence, based more often on hearsay than on the writer's personal experience. Nevertheless the alleged facts were presumed to derive from someone's observations, someone whose report was given full credence.

Unusual properties (or virtues) resident in particular objects are *occult,* that is, hidden from our senses, and their causes are not manifest. Such properties must in the first instance be discovered by experience. Agrippa declared very explicitly that these occult qualities whose causes are hidden can be reached only by long experience and not by exercise of the intellect or rational investigation.[25]

If we accept the general principle that many things possess occult virtues which can be identified through experience, then we have the task of somehow explaining these phenomena. That is, we must tie up the observations to acceptable concepts. The prevailing intellectual climate was Neo-Platonic, whose original principles and their partial degeneration we have already briefly discussed. The immediate problem now is how to apply the dominant philosophical concepts.

The occult virtues which inhere in things are comparable to the soul acting in a body. The essential virtues and powers derive from the celestial realm of Being, that is, from God. But any virtue, to proceed from God into the concrete world, must pass through a continuous chain of being, from God to Mind, from Mind to Soul, and from Soul eventually into body. This process, however, did not take place immediately. There was no automatic implantation of special properties into objects. Instead there was a creative or managing agent involved, the Demiurgos, or World-Soul (the very highest of the hierarchy of souls). The Demiurgos, who acted as foreman, so to speak, implanted the specific virtues into objects, but he did so *not directly but only through an intermediary way-station, namely, through the stars.* The stars were, in a sense, the *depot* for all specific properties and qualities. In this formulation every specific virtue came eventually from a transcendent God, but became specifically operative only after the Soul of the World first impressed them on the heavenly bodies and thence into earthly objects. "On the Stars, therefore, shapes and properties, all vertues of inferiour species as also their properties do depend."[26] The stars are *way-stations,* on the road from the Absolute Perfect One to earthly multiplicity and imperfection.

If we consider the heavenly bodies as intermediaries which link God to earthly things, then the movements, properties, and conjunctions of the stars and planets become very important. This is the theoretical basis of astrology, which depends quite directly on Neo-Platonic metaphysics.

The actual passage of celestial virtues into earthly things takes place by means of radiation. The "Seals and Characters" reside in the stars whose rays transmit these virtues. Of earthly objects, elements, stones, plants, and animals, each receives "from its Star shining upon it, some particular Seal or Character stampt upon it, which is the signification of that Star." Each particular object "hath its character pressed upon it by its Star for some peculiar effect, especially by that Star which doth principally govern it."[27]

There is, however, a further intermediate step between the Heavenly Ideas and concrete things. This intermediary, whose metaphysical status unfortunately involves some confusion, is the quintessence.

The term "quintessence" became prominent with Aristotle, who designated thereby a very special kind of material substance. The four elements, we recall, earth, air, fire, and water, had long been accepted as the material foundation of earthly things. But there was no evidence that they formed the objects beyond the earth. On the contrary, Aristotle maintained definitely that they did not. He believed that the earth was the center of the universe and was surrounded by a series of concentric layers. The inner layers were water, air, and fire. Beyond these were the celestial spheres which carried the sun, moon, and the planets, while the outermost sphere was that of the fixed stars. Heavenly bodies were incorruptible and unchanging, and quite perfect. Befitting their perfection was a composition quite different from that of the earth. The familiar four elements were not found. Instead, the spheres from the moon outward were composed of a fifth element, known as the *quintessence:* perfect, incorruptible, unchanging. It must be emphasized that the quintessence was material. It was not any sort of ideal entity, not an Idea or Form, but a very special kind of matter.

When, like Plotinus or Agrippa, we try to pass from a celestial world of divine intellect, ideas, and soul to reach a crudely material concrete world of here and now, the transition is not easy. Some special intermediary seemed necessary that might share in both worlds. Agrippa followed those of his predecessors, especially Marcilio Ficino (1433–99),[28] who believed that in addition to the soul there was a spirit which was finely material, and which could be the intermediary between soul and body. Agrippa specifically declared that the body was united to the soul by the spirit, while the understanding (or mind) was united to the spirit by the soul.[29] Thus, the spirit was a sort of ambiguous cement that could unite dissimilar entities.

Man and the world mirror each other. Just as man (the microcosm) has mind, soul, spirit, and body, which represent the progression from the ideal to the material, so too does the great world (or macrocosm) have its equivalents.

Corresponding to the microcosmic "spirit" there was, in the macrocosm, the "quintessence." Agrippa declared, "For as the powers of our soul are communicated to the members of the body by the spirit, so also the Vertue of the Soul of the World is diffused through all things by the quintessence."[30] It was, according to Ficino, "a very subtle body; as it were not body and almost soul. Or again, as it were not soul and almost body."[31] Agrippa adopted almost the identical words. The spirit was an intermediate essence, connecting the soul with the body, "quod sit quasi non corpus sed quasi iam anima, sive quasi non anima & quasi iam corpus, quo videlicet anima corpori connectatur," forming a "spiritum mundi" or "essentiam quintam."[32]

Thus, to bridge the gap between soul and body, between the ideal and material, there was invoked something which was neither, but which could nevertheless share the properties of both and serve as a connecting link. A concept of a material substance so fine and subtle that it was not really matter at all, was a very useful philosophical and theological device. From it arose the tradition of an "astral body" which the soul in its descent acquired before entering the world.[33]

These concepts indicate how severe was the difficulty under which the fifteenth- and sixteenth-century philosophers labored. As Neo-Platonists they could not accept the materialism which Stoicism represented. Yet while committed to a firm distinction between soul and matter, they could not pass satisfactorily from one to the other without some intermediary. Therefore they adopted the notion of something half-and-half, an astral body, a quintessence, a spirit which was material but not material. They did not appreciate how unsatisfactory is a *tertium quid* to connect dissimilars, but smuggled a Stoic metaphysics into their Platonism.

The Church had erected certain very rigid conceptual barriers, whose transgression meant heresy. Christianity held fast to the dualistic view, vigorously maintaining a distinction between an outside agent which provides activity, and that passive material on which the agent acts. The soul was the source of motion and activity. Therefore it had to remain completely distinct from matter. And conversely, matter without soul was completely inert. If matter could be self-moved, if activity were its inherent or intrinsic property, then the whole celestial realm might crumble into nothingness. At best a pantheism might remain, but this, of course, was anathema. Materialism, even in the ethically lofty form of Stoicism, was quite incompatible with Catholic doctrine.

Yet it was very difficult to pass from a transcendent immaterial force to inert matter. The solution which seemed acceptable achieved its success by bringing in certain Stoic (or materialistic) concepts *sub rosa*. From this point of view the quintessence and the astral body were subterfuges to avoid an otherwise insoluble problem, a problem which Descartes posed in all its stark difficulty.[34] The Renaissance thinkers had to bring in materialism covertly, while denying it openly.

The quintessence was significant for a further reason. It tended to supersede the Platonic ideas, and to take over their function. This was not a deliberate move in any sense, but came about gradually, as science developed, and as some form of materialism replaced idealism. While scholars may dispute the precise relation of Platonic "ideas" and medieval "substantial forms," yet viewed broadly they are equivalent. The substantial form of anything was its essence, "that which makes a thing what it is, and differentiates it from all other objects of the same genus. It is also called the specific form."[35] Such forms, existing as ideas in the mind of God, were eternal and

106

incorruptible. Eternal ideas in the mind of God were quite remote. They might serve as objects of contemplation, but scarcely as subjects of experiment. The quintessence also was perfect, unchanging, and incorruptible, but had the added advantages of dynamic activity and of proximity. You could (try to) get hold of a quintessence, wrest it from its covering, *do* something with it. As materialism covertly replaced idealistic dualism, the quintessence was a powerful weapon in the transformation. Unfortunately for the historian of ideas, there was much vagueness and considerable confusion attending the concepts, so that facile generalization must be avoided. But we may safely say that as empirical investigations flourished there was a swing away from ideas and forms toward the quintessence.

Compared with the mutable elements earth, air, fire, and water, the quintessence offered perfection, stability, permanence, and at the same time an intrinsic dynamic quality. In brief, it offered most of what an atomistic or materialistic formulation could provide, though within an orthodox framework.

Agrippa stressed the role of the stars in transferring "virtues" from the divine realm to the earthly sphere. This occurred through the quintessence or spirit, which "is received or taken in by the rayes of the Stars," and by it "every occult property is conveyed into Hearbs, Stones, Metals, and Animals, through the Sun, Moon, Planets, and through Stars higher than the Planets."[36] The concept of radiation, as known in the sixteenth century, seemed a splendid vehicle whereby something immaterial might affect something concrete.

Those who dealt with mundane things could achieve great advantage if only they could separate the quintessence or active virtue from the inert ingredients. If this were not feasible, it might be possible to identify those objects in which it most abounded, for objects with a greater proportion of activity, essence, or spirit would be more *effective* in satisfying practical needs. This search for the quintessence is the search for power, the search which underlies all magic, alchemy, divination, astrology, and all the so-called occult arts.

We must not speak of alchemy as if it were a single doctrine, or of alchemists as if they were a unified group. Actually, alchemical doctrines extended far into antiquity,[37] but we are now concerned only with the late medieval and Renaissance periods in Western civilization. The popular idea, that alchemy sought to change base metals into gold, using for this purpose something called the philosopher's stone, is misleading. Redgrove[38] declared that alchemy tried to demonstrate, in experimental fashion and on a material level, a certain philosophical view of the cosmos. Philosophy, we shall recall, was not merely contemplative. The alchemists were not content to meditate whether the universe was one, whether interconnections existed among things, but tried to apply their doctrines in concrete fashion. Those workers who kept close to practical and experimental techniques foreshadowed the chemists of a later age. But others "deserted their alembics and melting pots"[39] and devoted themselves chiefly to doctrinal points, to mysticism and speculation. Jacob Boehme (1575–1624) and Thomas Vaughan (1622–66) may be especially noted as mystics, for whom alchemy lost its practical or concrete significance and became merely symbolic. With mysticism as such we have no concern.

In earlier times, however, theory and practice were more intimately related. The theoretical aspects may seem to us quite fanciful but they represented a logical development from acceptable philosophical doctrine. From the practical standpoint alchemy concerned itself particularly with metals and the changes from one metal to another, or one element to another. Alchemical doctrine rested on observation. For example, the transmutation of what were considered to be elements was quite common. "By striking two hard stones together we produce fire; by boiling water, air is created; by the condensation of air, we obtain water; by the distillation of water, we become possessed of a residue of earth."[40] This latter phenomenon refers to the familiar observation that water boiled for a long time may show some "earthy" matter. At the same time transmutation in the organic sphere seemed equally clear. So-called "spontaneous generation" referred to the appearance of living creatures from the decomposed residue of dead creatures.[41]

The term "spirit," so widely used in occult literature, unfortunately bears many different meanings. The concept might be oriented toward material things, referring to special subtle components, or essence; or toward psychic, moral, and religious aspects. In any object the inward essence and the outer properties are comparable to soul and body. In order to secure the essence the outer shell must be peeled away. The spirit, the essence, the Truly Real, the celestial component filtering down from the stars, the effective and efficient mechanism inhering in an object (animate or inanimate)—all these were freely interchangable. Moreover, symbolism entered in and markedly confused a picture none too clear at best. Gold, for example, could be considered moral perfection with a spiritual beauty proof against evil. Lead, on the contrary, the "basest" of metals, represented sinful and unregenerate man. The philosopher's stone symbolized Jesus Christ. Transmutation was the regeneration of man effected by the spirit of Christ.[42] Such symbolic thinking obviously rendered very difficult any precise interpretation of observed phenomena.

Nevertheless we have a substantial germ of modern chemistry. There was an effort to strip off all impurities, secure the essence, modify it as necessary, and build up new substances. An important metaphysical implication is involved. As attributes were somehow peeled away, it was believed that substances would be reduced to prime matter as the ultimate. Matter in the Aristotelian sense represented pure potentiality, which under appropriate control might be reoriented toward a different actuality. The philosopher's stone, so-called, was the tool (or perhaps the term catalyst might be more significant) that would render this transformation easy. But even without the philosopher's stone, much progress might be made.

It is not our wish to analyze alchemy for its own sake. Thorndike[43] offers an indispensable exposition and critique, while Crombie,[44] Pagel,[45] Multauf,[46] and Taylor[47] may also be mentioned among the important secondary sources. For our purposes alchemy is significant insofar as it illustrates the general philosophy which furnished the background for Paracelsus.

In the realm of magic two types were distinguished. In demonic magic the results depended on personalized angels or demons as intermediaries. Incantations, prayers, talismans or figures, and acts of will were involved. On all of this the Church frowned. On the other hand was "natural" magic which acted impersonally, through natural forces and powers, the intrinsic properties of things, and planetary influences. No personalities, celestial or otherwise, were involved. This type of magic was deemed "good," especially if directed toward medicinal ends.[48]

There was no essential distinction between the major occult arts and the minor arts of divination, such as chiromancy, physiognomy, metaposcopy, pyromancy, oenomancy, and even umbilicomancy. These subjects all had a common belief: the connections among things were so intimate that *an observer by inspecting certain aspects of reality could find out a great deal about many other as-*

pects. Consequently the practitioners of these arts studied
the hand, the features, the lines of the forehead, the character of flames, the color and peculiarities of wine, and
even the properties of the umbilical cord at birth. These
all had special *meanings,* which the initiate could read.
Such beliefs, which numbered among their adherents
many acute intellects of the fifteenth and sixteenth centuries, were closely allied philosophically to magic. The
present-day palmist or tea-leaf reader is the lineal descend-
ant.

The numerous occult arts depended on a view of the
cosmos. Implied or expressed was a hierarchy of reality,
with interconnection of the celestial and the mundane. All
things, however, ultimately arose from God. There was
the notion of essence which might be manifested in outward properties. These outward properties might be regarded as signatures of the inner virtues.[49] In addition to
the essential qualities, there also existed "matter," which,
however, had variable meanings from the *hyle* of Aristotle
to the materialism of the Stoics, or of Lucretius. The concepts of process, activity, and function were important,
and the idea that the magician (or philosopher) may control function by penetrating to the essence and isolating it.
These are some aspects of the intellectual environment
from which Paracelsus developed his ideas.

IV

Within the compass of this book we can offer only
limited exposition of the doctrines of Paracelsus. Pagel's
recent studies[50] offer the most complete available analysis.
Our purpose is primarily to consider the ways in which
Paracelsus explained disease, and the explanatory concepts,
implicit and explicit, which he offered.

To begin with, all knowledge and all wisdom came

from God, who is the ground of all things. But the physician's dependence on God is metaphysical rather than religious. God is the source of existence and of nature, the guarantor of truth, the basis of wisdom. Nature is rooted in God (as is consonant with a Neo-Platonic philosophy), but there is no opposition between "natural" and "supernatural." Nature depends directly on God, and whoever thinks otherwise is in error. The physician, without God, is only a "pseudomedicus."[51] Nature, then, is the realm of the physician, but nature is also the realm of God who made it. Knowledge of God is knowledge of nature, and vice versa.

Medicine, then, the study of health and disease, is intimately involved with nature. Paracelsus indicated[52] that there were four columns of the medical art, four bases on which medicine rests. These were philosophy, astronomy, alchemy, and virtue, but only the first three need concern us. Philosophy, astronomy, and alchemy form a complex whole, no part of which can be understood without the others.

The first "column" is "philosophy." Although today this term usually connotes some type of speculative thinking, often contrasted to "science," Paracelsus did not intend any such opposition. On the contrary, "philosophy" for him clearly represented that activity which later came to be called "natural philosophy." This, of course, developed in turn into "natural science," and finally "science," unqualified. Philosophy for Paracelsus meant the study of nature. From nature arises not only disease, but the medicines to combat it. The physician, therefore, must study nature, the source both of disease and of remedies.

There are no sharp limits to philosophy. In general, those who study things of the earth are philosophers; of the heavens, astronomers. But the distinction is artificial because all things, heavenly and earthly, are interrelated.

The planets and stars, as we shall see, are intimately connected with things of this world. The astronomer knows
the fruits of the earth, and he knows Saturn and Jupiter;
and the philosopher knows the influence and course of
the heavens, the air as well as the earth. The astronomer
and philosopher know and judge the same thing. Despite
different names it is all one science. "Und wiewol da sind
geschiden namen, es seind aber nit geschiden kunst oder
geschiden wissen, das ist scientiae: dan eins ist in allen."[53]

In order to study medicine the physician must study all
knowledge. He must know about tin and copper, gold
and iron; must know what melts in lead, what liquefies
in wax, why diamond is hard, why alabaster is soft. Who
knows these things may then know how an abscess ripens,
what brings about the plague.[54] Thus the unity of all
knowledge is clearly indicated, the inner and true relevance of all things. Such a view, obviously, was not original with Paracelsus, but goes back to early Greek philosophy, and the concept of *physis*.

Paracelsus sought a rational basis for medicine. The
bases hitherto operative he believed were very inadequate.
Nothing less than the universe as a whole served as his
background. As if anticipating Francis Bacon, he took all
knowledge for his province. Indeed, the understanding
and cure of disease involved all knowledge, which he correlated with philosophy. Paracelsus distinguished fantasy
and imagination, which are based on false doctrine, from
truth, which is based on nature.

Paracelsus took a rather dim view of other people's
writings. Medicine, he believed, cannot be learned from
books, which are full of error. The only book we need is
the book of the firmament, which teaches according to the
light of nature, and which has its own alphabet. The stars
of the firmament make letters and sentences. The book of
the stars is free of deception, has written nothing falsely,

and need not be written on paper in order to be read. The book of the firmament, if put on paper, is like a shadow on the wall or an image in a mirror. If we really want to learn, we must see directly whence the shadow comes. That is, we must have direct experience.[55]

The study of the firmament and of the heavens, which he called astronomy, constitutes the second pillar or base of Paracelsian medicine. But "astronomy" must be understood in a rather special sense. There is no sharp distinction between things of the heavens and things of the earth. Nature is dependent on the heavens, and so are we who are part of nature. The great world, or macrocosm, includes the heavens, and only through its study can we understand the workings of the microcosm.

All things, declared Paracelsus, remain subject to the heavens and exhibit their will. Diseases derive from the heavens and remedies are managed and directed by the stars.[56] If we try to think of astronomy in any modern sense, Paracelsus' writings can only appear nonsensical. But if we regard "astronomy" as an element of Neo-Platonic philosophy, as already discussed, then his writings form a fairly logical and reasonably consistent whole. In our interpretation, the heavenly bodies represent the source of the "forms" or universals which terrestrial things exhibit. *The stars represent the Platonic forms or eternal relationships*[57] which, in Neo-Platonic fashion, become impressed on earthly things. The inner essences, the truly real, are derived from the stars, which in turn derive from God. To study the stars is to study the laws which govern things; correspondingly, when we seek the permanent laws and universal relationships which govern concrete objects, we are seeking the celestial properties, that is to say, the properties which are "in" the stars. The realm of the stars we would interpret as the realm of "natural law," into which the physician tries to penetrate. It is quite apparent that the study of books will not convey the insight that direct observations would yield, and we can see some point to Paracelsus' insistence that the physician can learn medicine only from direct observation of disease, and not from reading books.

As a philosopher, Paracelsus was not at all systematic. He did not try to analyze the problem of universals in any general sense, but was content to indicate that the stars had to do with complex relationships. They also had to do with the "spiritual" or "immaterial" aspects of things, the hidden properties and "virtues" which inhered in objects and which magic and alchemy disclosed. Paracelsus distinguished the visible, material, and corporeal from the immaterial, spiritual, and sidereal.[58] Everything that was dynamic had its sidereal aspect. The regularity and order of things, the predictability of events, all arose from dynamic properties which, in turn, derived from the spiritual and sidereal realm. The stars were connected with "spirit" and were intermediate between God and things.

This interpretation views Paracelsian "astronomy" as a Neo-Platonic legacy, very similar to the background on which Agrippa based his magic. We do not believe that Paracelsus in any way deliberately sought to transplant Neo-Platonic doctrine into medical theory; nor, probably, did he even see, let alone try to resolve, any of the attendant difficulties or inconsistencies. But he slipped into this mode of thought as a "matter of course."

If we interpret the heavens as the realm of essence and dynamism, law and regularity, as an intermediate station between God and the world, we have a serious problem very relevant to church doctrine. If celestial forces direct human affairs, what happens to free will? Latter fifteenth-century thought became much agitated over this point.[59] The stars may influence earthly activities. This is not heresy. But if the stars determine our actions, then free will is denied and we have heretical doctrine.

The way in which Paracelsus handled this problem, even though confused, is nevertheless quite significant. It is the heavens, he declared, which make things happen. The stars cause illness; they kill, and also cure. And what the heavens regulate and perform, they may announce, i.e., predict.[60] Nevertheless, he makes it clear that the stars do not determine events. "The stars do not control anything in us, they mold nothing in us, they do not irritate anything, they bias nothing; they are free by themselves and we are free by ourselves."[61] He is saying, in brief, that although the stars act on us, their action is not entirely conclusive.

If we interpret his statements broadly, in the light of what we have previously said, the contradiction may be resolved. If the stars are, figuratively speaking, the realm of order and "natural law" and "scientific necessity" (so-called), then the heavens control the sequences which medical science studies. Whereas we today would look to chemistry for the "laws" of, say, water-balance, Paracelsus invoked the activity of the stars. We might implicate aldosterone or antidiuretic hormone in explaining fluid balance. Paracelsus implicated Venus, the planet which controls the kidneys.[62] Just as the production and activity of adrenal secretions we believe are "determined," according to "laws" that we can discover, so the celestial bodies "made" things happen. The stars represented necessity. They determined *how* things happened, but *by themselves* they did not determine *whether* things would happen. *If* their activity applied, they determined the sequence of events, but it was not the stars *per se* which determined whether the activity *would* apply. The stars would determine the course of a disease, but would not indicate whether a given person would contract the disease.

116

The problem that haunted the sixteenth century was to exorcise the specter of rigid determinism, allow freedom of the will, and yet maintain validity for scientific "laws." We face the same problem today. Paracelsus, we believe, realized that there were in nature strict relationships and correlations, which were later called "laws." These predictable relationships which mundane things exhibited arose, he thought, from the celestial and sidereal realm. And indeed, in his philosophy, the celestial realm had no significant function other than to transmit into earthly things these very sequences and properties that were predictable.

The third pillar of medicine, intimately connected with the other two, is alchemy. Although alchemy in the popular imagination concerns the transmutation of metals into gold, this represents only one rather insignificant facet. Alchemy for Paracelsus concerned the general problem of change. We start out with one substance and end up with something quite different. How does it come about? The most striking examples are in biology. We plant a seed. A plant grows, yields fruit, and dies. We collect grapes and express the juice which then turns into wine. We take wheat and transform it into bread. We eat the bread which turns into flesh. If a man eats the bread it becomes human flesh. But the very same bread, if eaten by a pig, becomes pig's flesh. How does it all happen? These are very puzzling phenomena.

Greek philosophy, which tackled the problem, proposed several possible solutions. Anaxagoras, we recall (p. 60), suggested an answer that is especially significant. He maintained that all qualities and properties were infinitely small "seeds." All the properties which an object would eventually exhibit, all the things which it would eventually become, pre-existed as minute seeds within that particular object. Thus, if wheat were to become bread which in turn became flesh, there existed within the wheat the "seeds" of bread and the "seeds" of flesh. According to such a view "change" merely reveals what is there all the time. The wheat seeds are removed and the latent bread-seeds then predominate, but these in turn give way to the contained flesh-seeds. It is like a nest of boxes-within-boxes.

Paracelsus, however, conceived of change as much more dynamic. He too used the same example. The harvest is transformed into bread, which in turn is transformed into flesh and blood. These transformations he called alchemy. It was an alchemist who produced the change.[63] This alchemist has a difficult job and needs to exert very fine discrimination. For example, any food that is eaten contains some elements that are nutritious, others that are harmful. And there is considerable specificity. A cow can eat grass, but a man cannot. Ordinarily, snakes and lizards when eaten are poisonous. But the peacock, Paracelsus declared, can eat snakes or lizards and can separate the good from the poisonous. Other animals cannot do this. The pig can live on the excrement of other animals, for the pig can extract nutrition from what other animals have excreted.

How does all this come about? Paracelsus believed that God had appointed an "alchemist" for each animal, residing in the stomach. "He has appointed an alchemist for us to convert the imperfect which we have to utilize into something useful to us so that we may not consume the poison . . . but eliminate it from the good."[64] How does it happen that the peacock can eat poisonous snakes and yet not be harmed? Simply because the peacock has a very "subtle" alchemist, very skilful in separating the good from the harmful. Similarly with the pig. "The pig's alchemist extracts food even from the excrements, which man's alchemist has not been able to do, . . . there is no shrewder alchemist that will analyze food more minutely than the pig's alchemist."[65] God, declared Paracelsus, has brought it about that "there is a quality, an ability and dexterity such that by virtue of it the poison is sifted from the good at no injury to body and food."[86] Although the poison lies mingled with the good, the alchemist eliminates what is harmful.

At first glance this appears to be sheer redundancy. Once we note that an activity occurs, such as the transformations which take place during digestion, do we add anything when we invoke a special agent? Is it not comparable to a gremlin or the renowned "virtus dormativa"? Not entirely. Paracelsus did more than merely put a name on an observed function. *He related the function in question to certain other activities.* Alchemy in the stomach is comparable to the alchemy of a growing tree. Both are related to the fermentation of wine or the extraction of iron from its ore. In all these cases there is alchemy. The alleged presence of an alchemist as agent does render vivid the relationship, even if nothing else. It indicates that the activity in question involves the art of alchemy.[87] Through this link Paracelsus related the biological world to the inorganic, the processes of digestion with other processes of chemistry. To be sure, he gave no details, he did not talk about secretion of hydrochloric acid or digestive enzymes, but he did perceive a link between apparently dissimilar activities.

Specific details, for the most part, often did not interest him very much. He did appreciate that the process was very complicated and could go wrong in innumerable ways. But all was very vague and general. For health, man must have a fine alchemist "who does a good analysis with good instruments, vessels and passages of elimination." But, he went on, "it is indispensable that the heavenly bodies are well disposed together with all the other powers . . . there are . . . many accidents that can happen to the body which spoil, disrupt, befoul and pollute the instruments, vessels and passages of elimination and, perhaps, break and clog them up."[68] In factual terms all this says nothing more than, "There are many ways in which the digestive process can go wrong."

Synonymous with "alchemist" is "vulcan," who also conducts chemical procedures. Declared Paracelsus, "Alchimia ist ein kunst, vulcanus ist der künstler in ir."[69] The concept of alchemy involves transformation from one state to another. This transformation, however, is not blind or accidental but involves purpose or goal. Things do not merely happen, but they tend toward a certain end. Nature, or God, provides certain concrete objects but these, relative to man, are not complete. Man, through alchemy, must transform the initial or raw material into its ultimate form. Bread, for example, comes from God, but not in its finished form. The three alchemists, farmer, miller, and baker, bring about the transformation. "Brot ist uns beschaffen und geben von got, aber nit wie es von becker kompt, sonder die drei vulcani, der baur, der mülner und der becker die machen brot daraus."[70]

God created iron but not the objects made out of iron. The iron must be smelted and separated from the slag: this is alchemy. A tree grows: God creates the wood but he does not make charcoal. This requires alchemy. The raw material is something which exists for its own ends. Through the efforts of an archeus or vulcan, it is transformed or *completed* into something suitable for us. The finished particular object is something appropriate for us, rendered suitable for our needs. There is an end or goal involved and the alchemist, archeus, or vulcan is the agent which achieves it.[71]

Paracelsus liked to employ a triadic format to describe change. He liked the terms "prime," "intermediate," and "ultimate" matter. This means only that in any transformation we begin with a (relatively) raw product, progress to an intermediate stage, and end up with a (relatively) finished product. We must stress the concept "relative," since the finished product of one transformation may be the raw material for another. Thus, bread is a finished product relative to the baker's alchemy. But it is only raw material in the transformation leading to flesh and blood. Where bread is prime matter, flesh is the ultimate matter. This sequence, it should be noted, involves alchemy of the microcosm, whereas the change from wheat to bread was part of the macrocosm. But one mirrors the other.

Alchemy was especially important in preparing medicinal remedies. Medicines, to be truly effective, had a dual requirement. There was first of all the favor of the stars, the proper planetary influences. Unless the stars were favorable, medicines were of no avail. The separate parts of the body were each controlled by a separate planet, and there was thus a division of authority among the celestial bodies. What concerned the brain was directed by the moon; the spleen, by Saturn; the heart, by the sun; the kidneys, by Venus; the liver, by Jupiter; the gall, by Mars. Medicines for these organs did not function unless the planets so directed.[72] But while the stars were the directing force, the medicines must be made suitable for astral direction. The stars, he declared, cannot lift a stone. They can direct and utilize only what is volatile. Hence, to have effective medications, alchemy must prepare the essential ingredients. This requires that the physician must secure the pure essence, which was hidden within the shell of corporeal elements.[73]

Effective medicines must be in their purest form, so that their hidden virtues may become more readily manifest. This involves the quintessence (see p. 104) which Paracelsus defined very clearly. Consonant with the notion that everything grows and lives, the quintessence is a material substance extracted and separated from all impurities and "dead" material. Most pure and subtle, it is freed of all the crude elements. The quintessence comprises the inner nature and power, the virtue and medicinal qualities of any object, free of any harsh or foreign substance. The quintessence embraces the complexion, dynamic properties and characteristics of any object, and represents a spirit comparable to the spirit of life. In natural objects the quintessence is durable, but in humans it is not. From human flesh or blood no quintessence can be extracted, for the spirit dies.[74]

To strip off the dross and purify the essence, there were certain recognized alchemical techniques. These involved disintegration by heat in various degrees, sublimations, calcinations, solutions, extractions, distillations, and the like. The original substance was disintegrated and the extraneous elements removed. For example, to extract the quintessence of musk or other aromatic substances ("aromatibus"), Paracelsus advised placing the substance in a glass receptacle with almond oil. This is digested in the sun. The oil is then separated from the residue and mixed with rectified spirits ("vinum rectificatum") for six days, and then distilled over a bed of ashes ("per cineres"). The quintessence goes over with the alcohol ("brantwein") but the almond oil remains. Then the alcohol is distilled off on a water bath ("per balneum") and the quintessence remains behind in concentrated form, as an oil.[75] Darmstaedter comments that the process is unduly complicated, for alcoholic extraction alone would have been enough.[76] But it is apparent that Paracelsus, along with other early alchemists, had a significant grasp of chemistry techniques.

Nevertheless, even if alchemy can produce purified medications, or arcana, the stars must be favorable or the remedies will avail nothing. It is worth pondering for a moment how the stars exerted their effect. Logically there had to be some intermediary between stars and earth. The heavenly bodies were not isolated but were carried by the surrounding air ("luft" or "chaos") in the same way that the white of an egg surrounds and carries the yolk. The egg-white (chaos of the egg) is visible and palpable, but the chaos carrying the stars is invisible.[77] The heavenly bodies, planets, stars, and earth itself, all have their circumambient air. The stars act through this environment. Poisonous stars may pollute the air and then transmit the pollution to us, and good qualities are similarly transmitted. The "ens astrale," or power of the stars, "thus signifies the odor, vapor, exudation of the stars as mixed with air" and this may affect us unfavorably. "Any person who is thus by his very nature antagonistic to a particular vapor, falls sick. But he whose nature is not incompatible with it, derives no harm from it."[78]

Paracelsus called this environment the M ("Mysterium"). If this circumambient M exhibits unfavorable properties, then harmful results will follow. But these harmful properties originate in the stars. For example, cold "does not originate with the M, but from the heavenly body which possesses this property. . . . In the same way acts also the heat of the sun. . . . Just as these two, heat and cold, are two properties of some heavenly bodies bringing such things to pass, so there are others which make the M sour, bitter, sweet, sharp, arsenic and the like. . . ."[79] Elsewhere he gives an analogy of the relations between stars and chaos: "And in the same manner as water is brought to a boil by fire, the chaos is that which is boiled by the element of heaven. And just as the meat in water gives up its strength to the water, so the stars are like the meat and give up their strength to the afore-mentioned chaos."[80] However, we must remember that the stars, unlike meat, do not run out of "strength."

The stars, then, are the source of qualities and activities, while the atmosphere, the invisible environment, the M, is only the recipient and transmitter. Pagel points out that this Mysterium represents the "prime matter" of philosophers, "incomprehensible, without properties, form, colour, or elemental nature."[81] We would stress the role that Mysterium plays as a metaphysical substrate, whereby ideal properties become concretely manifest. In Neo-Platonic terms the stars, as way-stations from the divine intellect, impress their virtues and powers into the "air" and thereby exert these powers on earthly things and events. The air, in this sense, is a "receptacle" by which immaterial virtues are made manifest. This receptacle is by no means identical with either the "receptacle" in the *Timaeus,* or the *hyle* of Aristotle, but does suggest a certain degenerated kinship to both.

When Paracelsus discussed the miners' diseases, this chaos or air assumed a more concrete quality. Chaos or air is not only a metaphysical property but is also that which we breathe, "a food for the lungs in the same manner as the growths of the earth are food for the stomach."[82] In the mines this chaos may be harmful, for it is "ruled" by the minerals in the mines. Paracelsus clearly saw that various minerals, such as antimony, arsenic, or mercury, can cause disease by affecting the air which miners breathed. If minerals close at hand can, through the invisible chaos (air), induce changes in man—and this was an inescapable fact of observation—then it was not difficult to believe that distant stars, by affecting their chaos, could also influence us in comparable fashion. The minerals close at hand and the far-distant stars all fell into a unified pattern, and the chaos or air was a common feature, a unifying concept which tied together many disparate facts.

All this does not, unfortunately, indicate just how the distant stars control the action of medicines. Paracelsus firmly believed that this occurred, but he did not concern himself overmuch with intermediate steps, or detailed linkages.

We must not expect from Paracelsus either consistency or rigorous demonstration. He was essentially a poet and not a scientist or philosopher, but his poetical insights embodied current philosophy in an irregular fashion. The net result was not a systematic orderly doctrine, but rather a crazy-quilt patchwork which nevertheless has a delicate logic all its own.

Paracelsus, inclined as he was to metaphor and analogy, constantly emphasized the behavior of living creatures. He repeatedly discussed the growth and development of seeds, plants, and trees, the ripening of fruit, and similar biological phenomena. Yet, while in living beings we note the changes in form and configuration, we do not see the driving propulsive dynamic force which is responsible. Paracelsus distinguished the outer visible form which changes with the seasons from the inner active responsible essence which is constant. These inner active essences come from the stars, which represent the eternal. The inner driving forces are invisible but they induce a predictable course of development. Only the philosopher, thought Paracelsus, can appreciate the inward dynamic aspect.

Paracelsus compared diseases to the growth of trees.[83] With diseases, as with trees, we can readily note the form and configuration. To use modern terms, we can readily observe signs and symptoms. But these are only the outer aspects whose observation requires no great wit, whereas the inner invisible essence, which regulates activity and *causes* the disease (in the way that the seed produces the tree), is known only to the true physician.

This distinction between the inner essence and the outer form underlies Paracelsus' opposition to the humoral theory. The four cardinal humors, which are crudely material, we can readily observe. Yet these, whether excessive or deficient, are only manifestations of the disease. The true essence of the disease, dynamic and functional, is connected with nature as a whole and with the heavens. Emphasis on the humors neglects all this and stresses only the concrete and the immediately discernible. The humors come from the disease, not the disease from the humors. The snow does not make the winter, but the winter makes the snow.

This attitude, essentially vitalistic, emphasizes the role of process, time, development, pattern, interrelation of things and their reciprocal influences. It stresses a dynamic organizing activity, to which traditionally the word "soul" has been applied. Paracelsus takes a similar attitude toward disease, emphasizing pattern, growth, and organization. It was the "seed" which directed and brought about the pattern that we recognize as a disease.

V

If now we try to find out how diseases actually arise and what the specific mechanisms actually are, we note rather complicated doctrines. In his voluminous works Paracelsus discussed several different mechanisms, not all consistent with each other nor forming a unified whole. We can consider only certain selected aspects.

The doctrine that tartar is the source of disease combines observation and inference, fact and conjecture, in rather intricate fashion. Let us first examine some of the underlying data. Tartar or "Weinstein" is the stony deposit found in wine casks. It was supposed, somehow, to result from the process of wine-making, which involved fermentation and was considered to be a "vital" process. The term "tartar" (which was not invented by Paracelsus but is said to go back at least to Albertus Magnus)[84] represented precipitation generally.

In the absence of critical discrimination, many different kinds of precipitation were considered related and were all lumped together. Furthermore, they were associated with "vital" activity. Calcareous deposits of many different types do occur in various parts of the body: around the teeth, in the kidneys or bladder, as well as the gall bladder, lungs, and elsewhere. The living body, within which these deposits occurred, was constantly involved in "digestion" of one or another sort. This, of course, was one way of indicating what we today express by "metabolism." The process was perhaps most obvious in the mouth, which clearly breaks down and transforms food in a sort of digestion, quite distinct from the more complete gastric digestion. The deposit around the teeth, to which the name "tartar" is still applied today, was considered to be a by-product of this manifest digestion occurring in the mouth. By generalization, all tartar, all stony deposits within the body, were assumed to be similarly a by-product of digestion.

To achieve this generalization, Paracelsus had to collect all the data into one system, give them a common foundation and basic uniform etiology. To accomplish this he had to make great inductive leaps and go way beyond the limits of then available evidence. In so doing, he paid too much attention to superficial similarities and failed to distinguish important differences. When we criticize thus, we have at our command a knowledge of precise details which he did not possess, and we should not condemn him for not knowing what he could not know. His attempts to form a unified system are worth analyzing, as an example of sixteenth-century medical thinking.

We start with a sort of hylozoism. Everything in nature, even the so-called inanimate objects, lives and grows.

Everything is in process. Process implies growth and change of state. Whatever grows must have some nutrition. Nutrition requires digestion in order to separate the useful from the inert or harmful. "Alle ding wachsen und leben, darumb so sie nun essen müssen, so müssen sie ein magen haben und dieselbige kraft."[85]

Everything, then, requires "food," part of which is utilized. That part which is not utilized remains as stercor, dung, or excrement. In animals and humans, of course, that material which is not used is excreted as feces. In *things*, however, the non-utilized portions may remain. They may even become coagulated. Thus, he thought that pebbles in a brook represented the coagulated stercor from the water, while mountain rocks ("bergstein") were the coagulated residue from the earth's nutriment.[86] "Natural things," although they take in nutrition as do animals, unlike animals cannot eliminate the useless portions, which therefore remain. "Scheidet . . . nit der natürlichen dingen stercus."[87]

It follows, therefore, that whatever man eats or drinks has a twofold composition: its own stercor and its own proper substance. This latter the human body can digest, utilizing what is nutritious and excreting the remainder as feces. But *the stercor of the food itself* the human body cannot selectively eliminate. In other words the *excrement of things we eat* remains attached to the food when we eat it, and represents a source of trouble.

The excrement of things we eat constitutes tartar, and is an undesirable material. How does it happen that some persons have tartaric diseases, others not? Paracelsus had to find some differential criterion. He relied on an old concept, namely, the "force" of digestion. Those who have a "weak digestion" do not sufficiently break down the food, so that bad material is eliminated unchanged. This might be something like a present-day "malabsorption syndrome" wherein tartar in "conjugated form" passes out unchanged and unabsorbed. But those who have a "strong digestion" break up the food more completely. The tartaric substances are thus liberated, and since they are not excreted, either remain in the gastrointestinal tract or are absorbed into the veins.[88] The tartar, which cannot be utilized, remains in the body without becoming part of it. Paracelsus does not explain just why the tartar cannot be excreted in human feces. This remains one of his assumptions.

It should be further mentioned that, as a differential feature to explain the incidence of tartaric diseases, Paracelsus recognized the intrinsic differences among foods. Clearly some foods were richer in this stercor than were others, so that a bad diet could induce tartar. The regulation of diet (the selection of "proper" foods) was therefore one way of controlling these diseases.

In "natural things" the excrements or stercors which constitute tartar may take four different forms, namely, stone, sand, clay ("letten"), and slime ("leim," indicating gelatinous, gluey, or mucinous substances). Stercor of things differs from stercor of man. Whereas in man the ultimate state of excrement is putrefaction, in things the excrement does not putrefy. Instead, its ultimate state is coagulation. The slimy and clayey components can become stony in character and be precipitated as tartar. The tartar does not simply "happen" in the tissues but is precipitated by an active agent, the "spirit of salt," which coagulates the tartar and transforms any mucilaginous or viscid material into stony substances.[89]

Paracelsus indulged in some interesting reasoning, based on particular assumptions. He argued from the known to the unknown. In the mouth we find tartar around the teeth; we also find various irritations, decay, aches and pains, or other kinds of "acrimony" in relation to the teeth, jaws, or oral cavity generally. The tartar, which we observe, is considered to be the "cause" of the pains and inflammation, which we also observe. This is a not unreasonable assumption. In other parts of the body we also find calcareous deposits, as in the kidneys, urinary bladder, or gall bladder. These quite manifestly are associated with severe pains, inflammations, and disabilities, for which also the "stone" can reasonably be adduced as cause. But then Paracelsus assumed the converse, that the existence of various other inflammations, pains, disabilities, and "acrimonies" generally, all indicated the presence of tartar. And if tartar could not be demonstrated visually, it could be assumed to be present in invisible form. Paracelsus was quite accustomed to accepting invisible causes for manifest phenomena.

He believed that tartaric deposits in stomach and intestine produce constipation and colic. In the intestine, he claimed, tartar may become so heaped up that nothing can pass and no purges or clysters can clear the passages.[90] This occlusion or obstruction presumably refers to carcinoma, which is often very hard, develops slowly, and of course is not relieved by purgatives. Here again we have uncritical inference, that because tartar was hard, anything hard was tartaric. A hard consistency, such as we find in many cancers and other sclerosing lesions, was assumed to indicate a form of tartar.

It was not too difficult to explain intestinal disease as tartaric manifestations. Pathogenesis appears relatively simple. Tartaric substances are swallowed; instead of being eliminated they are deposited, and then wreak their damage. But the tartars found in other bodily systems represent a more complicated pathogenesis involving basic physiological assumptions.

Digestion occurs in the stomach. The digested material, with its contained tartar, is absorbed from the stomach into the mesenteric veins, where nutriment is separated from waste. The waste material is urine. Paracelsus declared dogmatically, "Scheit sich der urin von dem nutriment in den meseraischen aderen und meatibus."[91] Tartar may be deposited within these mesenteric vessels, and, if in sufficient amount, may actually impair further absorption from the stomach. If this occurs, food may remain unabsorbed in the stomach and lead to vomiting. It is an interesting concept that vomiting could result from blockage of absorptive channels.

The mesenteric vessels, containing both nutriment and urine, pass into the liver. Ordinarily the liver draws off its own proper nutrition, and what is left proceeds toward the urinary passages. However, tartar may be deposited in the vessels of the liver substance and give rise to liver diseases. Among these Paracelsus specifically mentioned dropsy ("wassersucht").[92] It is noteworthy that he associated certain cases of ascites not only with liver disease generally but with disease of hepatic vessels specifically. This anticipates the concept that ascites may result from impaired portal circulation.

Urine, then, which was produced in the mesenteric veins, passes through the liver. The subsequent anatomical pathways are not made clear. Paracelsus declared that urine passing to the bladder has "etliche weg" from liver to kidneys, but these ways are not clarified. He had very little interest in anatomy, unfortunately, but he did believe that the urine was conducted to the kidneys, somehow. Tartar might be deposited anywhere along the path. As the urine approached the bladder, it became more ripe and mature, comparable to the ripening of a pear. But as the urine became more purified, any tartar which might be deposited in the excretory paths became sharper and stronger. Various symptoms then resulted, including pains, phlegmons and abscesses.[93] Presumably he developed this theory to explain why stone is more prominent in kidneys and bladder than in the mesenteric veins or liver.

These examples illustrate the action of tartar as a causative agent in disease. In the *Opus Paramirum,* Paracelsus discussed many other diseases due to tartaric substances, but detailed consideration would carry us far afield. Although tartar was considered a major cause of disease, it was not the only factor. We must also note the role of the air or chaos, and of the three elements.

When Paracelsus discussed the miners' diseases, he became much more concrete and practical and rather less philosophical than in other discussions. He dealt with concrete events that he had experienced. His observations were sound, his interpretations interesting.

Miners' diseases ("bergsucht") were part of pulmonary diseases generally ("lungsucht"). The lungs feed on air, "and as it is possible that food produces disease, thus it is also possible for the air to give birth to these things [disease]."[94] The air, or chaos, which lies between heaven and earth "produces all the diseases of the lungs, their fevers, ulcers, consumption, plethoras, cough, gasping, and oppression together with all the other kinds." As we have seen, the chaos is "governed" by the stars which affect the surrounding air, just as meat affects the water in which it is boiled. The stars, he said, produce a "soup," either healthy or unhealthy.[95]

The stars, then, are considered the active agents which affect the air, and it is the air which affects the lungs, for better or worse. Now the ordinary atmospheric air lies between the earth and the heavens. (Of course, Paracelsus had no notions regarding the limits of the atmosphere.) But within the mines there was a different chaos, which was regulated not by the stars but by the minerals of the mines. This earthly chaos affected the lungs of the miners and produced "mine-sickness" ("bergsucht"), whereas the more generic "lung-sickness" ("lungsucht") came from the heavenly (atmospheric) chaos. The different lung diseases have a similar pathogenesis. The air (chaos) of the mines "becomes a soup of its minerals in the same manner as the external chaos is a soup of the stars."[96]

Paracelsus clearly recognized that variations in the air we breathe produce various illnesses. To the "fog" which lies between heaven and earth he attributed "asthma, coughing, and short-windedness," while the "fog" in the mines caused the miners' diseases.[97] The minerals acted through this fog. That various minerals could cause disease was clearly known. Arsenic, for example, or antimony, was recognized as a poison if ingested. Paracelsus pointed out that the vapors which escape from an ore are also poisonous but with much diminished intensity. These poisonous vapors, which he called the "spiritus" of the mineral, could produce serious symptoms, but much more slowly than the "corpus" of the mineral (the solid substance). Whereas, for example, a dose of arsenic could kill in ten hours, the "spiritus" (acting through the lungs) would require ten years. And Paracelsus gave fine clinical descriptions of the symptomatology of chronic poisoning.[98] In his treatise he took up quite admirably the clinical aspects of various metallic poisons. Rosen[99] has presented an excellent analysis and appreciation.

At this point it is necessary to discuss the famous doctrine of the three "elements" which played such an important role in Paracelsus' theories. In his usage, "mercury," "sulfur," and "salt" did not at all correspond to the substances bearing these same names today. Paracelsus, in fact, was describing not objects but functions or properties which inhered in objects. These properties might not be at all apparent in a particular object. Take, for example, a piece of wood. The wood will burn, it gives off smoke, and leaves an ash as a residue. These are the properties of wood which are truly significant. What burns is "sulfur"; what goes off in smoke is "mercury"; what remains as ash is "salt." These represent the basic properties or components of matter: a combustible portion, a volatile portion, and an inert or resistant portion. These properties inhere in all things, and if not immediately evident are readily demonstrable through science. Moreover, it is only sulfur which burns, only mercury which sublimes, and only salt which constitutes residues.[100]

It follows that the mercury in one substance is not the same as the mercury in another. Since each object has its own mercury, sulfur, and salt, there are as many different kinds of these "elements" as there are classes of objects.[101] This viewpoint stresses the dynamic aspect of things, and indicates the emphasis on function rather than structure. It is what an object does which was important to Paracelsus. The term "element" meant a basic or irreducible function. The material components or building-blocks were not very important.

Paracelsus might use the same terms in rather varied senses, but the most common meaning of "sulfur," for example, was simply something which burns. Substances of widely different character might all possess the quality of combustibility and, neglecting all differences, might be construed as similar. In lung diseases, for example, Paracelsus indulged in a devious chain of inference. Certain characteristics of the lung which he called resinous (possibly referring to caseation?) he considered to be a "sulfur." This resinous material came from a sulfur in the chaos, and this in turn came from the minerals which ruled that chaos. And the chaos is "furnished with a fixed sulphur. If this sulphur is seized by the lung, it attaches itself to the latter like a resin to a tree; this resin is the complaint and the cause of the miners' disease," for the lung cannot "digest" this sulfur in the chaos.[102]

In the chaos there is not merely sulfur (that is, the oily and resinous components) but also the volatile element called mercury. Each mineral has its characteristic sulfur and also its own mercury. Thus we have "a mercury of copper, a mercury of lead, a mercury of ore which has already been roasted, a mercury of zinc, a mercury of arsenic and the like."[103] And the chaos also contains a salt of each metal. These were all significant in pathogenesis, for Paracelsus believed that there were three chief types of miners' sickness. The spirit of sulfur produces a resin in the lung, the spirit of mercury yields a soot, and the spirit of salt, a tartar.[104] If we try to transpose these into modern pathologic equivalents, we might suggest caseation, anthracosis, and calcification, three conditions very common among miners.

Fire is the agent which separates a body into its components. In the smelting of ore, for example, the sulfur and mercury of that metal would be liberated. The mercury, or smoke, mixed with the air, is especially poisonous. When it enters the lungs it produces a variety of changes.[105] Paracelsus discussed at considerable length the separate metals and ores and the symptoms and bodily changes which they induced. He clearly perceived that various diseases resulted from products which, during the mining or smelting processes, came from the metals. How such emanations occurred, and how they wreaked their damage, he explained through his theories of mercury, sulfur, and salt. The modern reader, however much he may reject the theory, cannot but be impressed by the keen observations and accurate descriptions.

The mining and purification of metallic ores induced diseases in the miners, and the responsible agents were transmitted through the air. Paracelsus avoided any simple atomistic explanation. It might seem quite "obvious" that minute particles, minute atoms, of this or that metal, became separated off from the metal and floated into the air. This, however, is a simple "structural" explanation, and Paracelsus had very little interest in structure or anatomy. On the contrary, he was concerned first of all with function, activity, and behavior. And he was also concerned with tying together as many different kinds of activity as possible. It was important for him to know that a substance was volatile under certain conditions but not under other conditions. It was also important for him to relate the volatility of one agent with other examples of volatility in quite different areas. But what concrete structural element might be present was not important. Any atoms or minute particles were far removed from direct observation, and were only speculations and hypotheses that did not interest him.

The concepts of mercury, sulfur, and salt served as explanatory terms which could tie together quite varied data of observation in chemistry, metallurgy, and biology. Combustion, distillation, precipitation, solubility and insolubility, and vaporization, which we find in chemical reactions, he could relate to each other and to "resins" and "soot" and "tartar" in the body. Agents were at work, agents outside the body which could enter the body and produce disease, agents which obeyed certain regularities, whose behavior could be observed in many different modalities. All this, which is largely empirical, is significant. Paracelsus was quite ruthless with any theory which did not take account of these facts. He was particularly violent against the traditional humoral theories and the medical practice based thereon.

The more we study Paracelsus, the more we are able to overlook his bizarre terminology and appreciate his insights. He was not a physician who sought merely empirical cures, or who practiced medicine by rote, but was at heart a philosopher, trying to understand the universe and the connections between things. He disregarded surface appearances to seek a deeper underlying reality. The problem of reality, one of the great philosophic questions, has received many answers, but somehow, no matter what solution has been proffered, refuses to remain solved. Paracelsus adhered largely to the Platonic tradition, although quite variously modified. Unlike many important Renaissance figures, Paracelsus was not a classical scholar, and he did not go back to the original Greek texts. The various Platonic and Neo-Platonic doctrines, together with the Stoic overtones, he probably acquired at second- or even third-hand. Yet he found in them a dynamic formulation that he could apply to medicine and medical problems in the broadest sense.

We might say, perhaps, that the intellectual environment was very heterogeneous, showing many different elements; that Paracelsus perceived and elaborated certain particular trends, especially those in the Platonic traditions; that he modified this tradition in the light of his own experience and neglected or even condemned all other trends. He observed phenomena, considered their relationships, noted the connections, analogies, and similarities. But unfortunately he all too often neglected manifest differences. And this neglect impaired his scientific stature. It was not easy to acquire a severely critical attitude.

The observations and insights of Paracelsus ran counter to materialism. Actually, the materialistic approach led to very substantial progress in both theory and practice, so much so that the opponents of materialism seemed guilty of being false prophets and of following false gods. Nevertheless Paracelsus' insights were to bear fruit even after centuries of abuse. Later critics could separate the chaff from the grain and could properly evaluate this insight: to have realized that simple mechanical explanations are severely inadequate; to have related the organic and the inorganic through what we now call chemistry; to have appreciated the dynamic qualities of things and the inter-relation of events; to have grasped the basic Platonism of science, even though disguised or modified—these are a few of the merits of Paracelsus.

Progress and Pitfalls

VESALIUS, HARVEY, HOFFMANN

Paracelsus developed his concepts from a matrix of Greek philosophy, but his doctrines repelled those of a more prosaic mold who were concerned with the concrete rather than the abstract. In the Renaissance there was a sharper focus on the empirical world, a stronger tendency toward precision; observations became more accurate, discrimination more readily accomplished. New observations induced new theory—which reciprocally induced still further observations—to achieve a very fruitful cross-fertilization. The sixteenth and seventeenth centuries witnessed the rise of modern physical science, the growth of modern scientific method, the development of a "mechanical philosophy" and a mechanistic attitude. The story, with all its dramatic achievements, has been well described in many excellent recent studies.[1] It is not our purpose to trace in any way the growth of astronomy or physics, or to touch on the Cartesian or Newtonian philosophies. However, study of a few medical figures may indicate the manner in which medicine progressed along with the physical sciences.

To indicate the development of mechanistic doctrine in medicine we will start in the early Renaissance. Paracelsus was not typical of his era. If we would appreciate the more usual modes of medical thought and practice, we can do no better than to dip into the writings of Antonio Benivieni (1443–1502), whose book, *The Hidden Causes of Disease,* was published posthumously in 1507.[2]

This volume is a collection of case reports which in the aggregate vividly portray the medical environment in the early sixteenth century. Clearly revealed, although often indirectly, are the problems facing the practitioner, and the factors considered significant. Far from giving us a discrete medical philosophy, Benivieni seemed to relegate medical theory to a subordinate position. As we might expect in any highly empirical practice, there is no discussion of basic rationale behind the treatments. There is no articulate world-view such as we find in Paracelsus. On the other hand, the observations and descriptions are often sharp and clear. There is straightforward narration, and despite the hazy theoretical background we get an impression of honest recording. This is what he saw, this is what he did, this is what happened to the patient. To be sure, he accepted as fact much that we cannot accept. There is a large proportion of what we would call superstition, and a great deal that we would regard as simple credulity. Hence, while admiring his honesty we must often condemn his reports as uncritical.

For example, a young man suffering from a swollen knee, unsuccessfully treated by surgery, consulted Benivieni, who recommended cautery. This the youth refused, but, "despairing of medical skill, he fled to divine aid," via a Dominican monk. Through the latter's prayerful ministrations the "malady was completely removed within a few days," and Benivieni himself testified that the knee was entirely sound.[3] He also described cures supposedly achieved through necromancy.[4]

But despite such lapses from what we would consider scientific method, Benivieni recorded many cases with straightforward simplicity. He described many successful surgical operations. He cured cases of vaginal and of anal atresia.[5] An ulcer of the chin he considered to be due to a decayed tooth, and by removing the offending tooth achieved a cure. A swelling of the leg, whose nature is not clear but which he called "elephantiasis," he successfully treated by excising the fibula.[6] He recorded many post-mortem findings which, even though no proper therapeutic means were at hand, indicated accurate observation. Mention may be made of patients who had undoubted carcinomas of intestines and stomach.[7]

When we have description without excessive concern with theory, we have a background suitable for medical progress. The medical practice which is content to observe and record has the merit of avoiding dogmatism, and there may be a receptiveness to new observations—and to new theory—which would not obtain in a stiff-necked doctrinaire. Benivieni seems to have been essentially a simple empiric, who by open-mindedness invited progress.

II

During the sixteenth century medical progress occurred largely through anatomy, a subject which demands straightforward and precise observation, yet does not require much theoretical elaboration. However, the study of anatomy before the Renaissance was largely held in check by authority, namely the authority of Galen, whose writings had attained canonical status.

The study and teaching of anatomy underwent great changes during the Renaissance, changes which contemporary documents graphically exhibit. In 1493 there was published a collection of older anatomical tracts translated into Italian. The longest of these, the *Anathomia* of Mundinus (1270–1326), superbly illustrates the conduct of an early dissection. The picture, reproduced in Singer,[8] and Singer and Rabin,[9] shows the anatomist, the "professor." From his "chair," an elevated structure well above the cadaver, he would read aloud from a book. Meanwhile the actual dissection was performed by a menial, called a *demonstrator*. Such a person needed some degree of dexterity perhaps, but not any real knowledge of anatomy. Intermediate between the professor and the man who dissected was a third person, the *ostensor,* who with a short staff or wand pointed out the actual structures as the knife-wielder exposed them, and as the professor described them from a book. We find essentially the same procedure illustrated as late as 1535, in Berengario da Carpi's *A Short Introduction to Anatomy ("Isagogae breves")*.[10] In neither case did the students who crowded around the body participate in the actual dissection. They were merely spectators.

Vesalius himself described the methods previously in vogue, wherein one man dissects while another reads the description. "These latter are perched up aloft in a pulpit like jackdaws, and with a notable air of disdain they drone out information about facts they have never approached at first hand, but which they merely commit to memory from the books of others . . . [;] the former [the dissectors] are

142

so ignorant of language that they are unable to explain their dissection to the onlookers and botch what ought to be exhibited in accordance with the instruction of the physician, who never applies his hand to the dissection, and contemptuously steers the ship out of the manual, as the saying goes. . . . In the confusion less is offered to the onlooker than a butcher in his stall could teach a doctor."[11]

However, new ideas and methods were taking form. In 1531 a Latin translation of a Galenic text was published, the title page of which illustrated a dissecting scene[12] that is rather different. The lecturer stands at the head of the table, but no books are in evidence, nor do we see any *demonstrator* or *ostensor*. Instead, enthusiastic students are handling and even passing around the organs. This scene may be considered transitional to the modern procedure, so magnificently portrayed as the frontispiece of Vesalius' *De fabrica* (1543), wherein the teacher not only lectures but performs his own dissections and demonstrations.[13]

Vesalius, more than any other single figure of the sixteenth century, helped transform medicine from medieval to modern form. It is perhaps an overstatement to say that his *De humanis corporis fabrica* "established with startling suddenness the beginning of modern observational science and research,"[14] for no great movements can be attributed solely to one individual or one work. Nevertheless, if in a brief survey we wish to indicate the transition to modern medicine, we can do no better than consider Vesalius and then Harvey.

In fifteenth-century medicine, anatomy occupied a rather peculiar position. It was a recondite subject. Physicians had to spend considerable time mastering the intricate details that Galen, the Arabian commentators, and others had described. These details were largely wrong. Nevertheless, wrong or right, it was knowledge of these details

143

which helped to distinguish the learned from the ignorant. Medical theory was to a large extent founded on anatomy. Yet if we look backward quite dispassionately, we must ask how much practical difference it made whether the anatomical information at that time was strictly correct. The learned physicians treated internal diseases. The therapeutic tools at their command were indeed scanty. Can we really believe that knowing an accurate description of the liver, or the true course of the veins or the arteries, would have enabled Benivieni to treat his patients any more effectively? In the medical environment then obtaining, an accurate anatomical knowledge was not practically useful for physicians.

Surgery was largely split off from medicine and handed over to the barbers. Vesalius greatly regretted this split, and declared that, "When the doctors supposed that only the care of internal complaints concerned them, they neglected the structure of bones and muscles, as well as the nerves, veins and arteries which run through bones and muscles, as of no importance to them."[15] And so dissection, he declared, soon died out. Vesalius might have added that in Paris at this time, those physicians who became licentiates of the Faculty of Medicine "promised solemnly to adhere to the statutes of the College, including that which forbade them indulging in the practice of Surgery or Anatomy, or any manual craft—for the dignity of the profession was dependent on this ban."[16] This was indeed a slightly schizophrenic attitude. In Paris the study of anatomy was apparently regarded as merely an obstacle course. When you had passed the obstacle and achieved high medical status, then to preserve the "dignity" of your guild, you were forbidden to investigate the subject further. It must be noted, however, that bachelors of medicine, who had not yet become licentiates, could study anatomy at first hand.

Anatomy is very important, practically, for surgeons. Yet considering the surgical techniques then available, we might still question whether a more precise knowledge of osteology or muscle-insertions would have made any significant difference. All too many surgeons were profoundly ignorant even of the imperfect anatomy then available. There was already at hand considerable information which, though not entirely accurate, would nevertheless have been eminently serviceable had it been more widespread.

However, when we question how much concrete difference a correction of Galen would have made, either in everyday medicine or everyday surgery, we are facing only one aspect of the problem. The appeal of anatomy, we must recognize, is twofold. There is a certain practical aspect within which high accuracy is not very important. "Accurate enough" is allowable.

But anatomy exerts another appeal, apart from practical advantages. There are those who seek precision for its own sake, who want to acquire exact knowledge merely for the sake of knowing. These are pure investigators; what they study is pure science. For the scientist error must not be tolerated, even though the correction of that error does not now make much practical difference. Truth, not practical benefit, is the touchstone. Vesalius was one who sought knowledge for its own sake.

We must not for a moment believe that Vesalius single-handedly established modern medical science. It is sometimes held that publication of the great *De fabrica* in 1543 marked a break with the Galenic tradition, that the Galenists were bigots, that Vesalius overthrew the prevailing Galenic teachings and established a new scientific approach. This view has been vigorously attacked by recent scholars[17] who have traced the development of anatomical studies prior to Vesalius and have indicated the scientific achievements of his predecessors and contemporaries. It is wrong to picture the Galenists as rather stupid reactionaries, and Vesalius as the liberator who struck off the shackles of error. Instead, as Montague declared, the *De fabrica* was not so much a break with Galenic tradition as an advance upon it.

There are many accounts of Vesalius' life,[18] so that only a few details need be recounted here. The highlights are well known. Born in 1514 in Brussels, he came from a long line of medical forebears, and his was the fifth successive generation of physicians. He acquired his preliminary education at Louvain, and in 1533 began to study medicine at the University of Paris where he came under the influence of Jacobus Sylvius (1478–1555) and Johannes Guenther (or Guinterius or Winter, 1487–1574). In 1536, because of war, he left Paris and returned to Louvain where he studied further as well as taught. In 1537 he went to Padua; there he took his doctor's degree, and became professor of surgery and anatomy. The *Tabulae anatomicae sex,* appeared in 1538 and the *De fabrica* in 1543. For reasons which are still not clear, Vesalius then gave up anatomy to join the court of Charles V and later that of Philip II. Yet apparently he was not happy. In 1564 he returned to Italy but died while on a pilgrimage to Jerusalem.

Vesalius was not a very lovable individual. He was splenetic, prejudiced, ungenerous, quick to take credit to himself, loath to give credit elsewhere. His judgments of his contemporaries and predecessors are quite unreliable. Recent scholars have helped to restore a suitable perspective. The *De fabrica* is indeed a work of genius, but we must recognize that it developed in an environment that others had already made favorable.

We must not believe that up to the time of Vesalius Galen's every word was slavishly accepted, or that anatomists regarded only the printed page and failed to observe for themselves. Berengario da Carpi, for example, noted Galenic errors that the medieval Mundinus had already corrected. And as for himself, Carpi declared that he accepted Galen's views except where observation was at variance therewith; and he warned that readers should not be deceived "by some of our moderns who involve anatomy with authorities and not with observation."[19] Sylvius, whom Vesalius roundly condemned, insisted on an empirical approach, in learning by doing rather than mere passive acceptance. He declared, "For my judgment is that it is much better that you should learn the manner of cutting by eye and touch than by reading and listening," and he stressed learning "by the use of one's own sight and the training of one's own hands."[20] In fact, Galen himself had declared that whoever wishes to regard the works of nature should not believe books but rather his own eyes.[21]

All this may seem mere lip service, honored in the breach rather than the observance, but the principle deserves some examination. All students of nature, ancient, medieval or modern, have relied on observation. Yet when personal experience disagrees with what others have written or declared, there may arise a conflict whose resolution is not easy. Tradition and authority are not lightly to be disregarded. What, for example, would we say to an elementary chemistry student whose experiment came out quite differently from the book? Quite obviously the student has made a mistake. His observation is not "correct." Nor do we believe our eyes when we "see" the sleight-of-hand artist restore a torn paper or make a coin vanish. Hippocrates had already noted that experience is deceptive. On the other hand, it is quite possible that a given observation or experience *is* "correct" even if it does contradict authority. In such a case the authority or tradition is wrong. But how, in a conflict between experience and tradition, are we to tell which is right? There are no rules that we can give to resolve any such conflict.

It is not enough to advise sagely to "study nature" or "rely on experience." The observer must have some way of evaluating his observation. It is all very well to tell a student to trust his own eyes, but this does not tell him how much attention to pay to what he sees, or how to evaluate what he sees compared to what he is told. If, on the basis of what he has seen, the observer is to disregard a contradictory authority or tradition, some new factor above and beyond a copy-book maxim is needed. There must be a flash of insight, of conviction, of assurance—and frequently of courage.

Vesalius, more than any other early sixteenth-century figure, achieved this insight and conviction, but he was not alone. In the first half of the sixteenth century important and progressive anatomists made new observations in a scientific manner. Berengario, Sylvius, Massa, Estienne, have received critical appreciation from modern scholars.[22] Indeed, the anatomist Fallopius declared in 1561, "The work that Berengario started, Vesalius completed."[23] It is worthwhile reviewing some of the steps that led from the Galenic tradition to the *De fabrica* of 1543.

In 1536 in Paris, Johannes Guenther published a little book which summarized some Galenic teachings. Guenther, probably never a skilled dissector, was nevertheless a profound classical scholar. His book, *Institutiones anatomices secundum Galeni sententiam*, was a brief survey in whose preparation the assistance of Vesalius, as well as of Servetus, was acknowledged. Guenther attributed to Vesalius the discovery of the origin of the seminal arteries and veins, a "discovery" which was already familiar to Massa, Berengario, and Mundinus.[24] Vesalius even as a student was a very skilful dissector, doubtless far superior to most professors, but we must realize that he was still very much a follower, not an innovator.

When Vesalius left Paris, he went first to Louvain and then to Padua. In 1538 he published two important complementary works. One was a revision of his teacher's *Institutiones,* for he had found through his own dissections and experience that this text needed correction. However, as Fisch declared, "The corrections were conceived as corrections not of Galen but of Guinter [Guenther]." His changes were not offered as innovations, but he "used his own observations to restore the sense of what he took to be corrupted passages."[25] In other words, in case of discrepancy between observation and authority, it was not Galen who erred but only his transcribers. This was one way of resolving any conflict between tradition and personal experience.

Vesalius' other publication in 1538 was the remarkable *Tabulae anatomicae sex,* analyzed at length by Singer and Rabin,[26] to which the *Institutiones* was essentially a companion piece. The *Tabulae* were six large anatomical charts, each with descriptive labels and brief comments. These charts, now called "fugitive pieces," were designed as student aids rather than as scholarly productions. They indicate what Vesalius believed in 1538. The first plate shows the liver and portal system and the organs of generation; the second the venous system (other than the portal); and the third the heart and arterial system. These three Vesalius himself drew. They are frankly Galenic, and contain numerous errors that reflect Galen's teachings. The last three plates depict a skeleton that Vesalius had prepared, seen from the anterior, lateral, and posterior positions. These, drawn by John Stephan Calcar, a pupil of Titian, are also not free from anatomical error derived from Galen.

In 1539 Vesalius published a small work on bloodletting, part of a dispute regarding the appropriate loci for therapeutic venesection. Here he insisted on the importance, the primacy, of personal observation. "It is in this small work," declare Saunders and O'Malley, "that we first perceive the slow and gradual loosening of traditional and authoritative bonds whence eventually emerged the principle that the validity of a hypothesis rests solely on the facts established by observation"[27] (p. 18). This letter on bloodletting is generally considered transitional to the *De fabrica* which appeared in 1543.

This masterpiece has been so widely discussed that here it is only necessary to note two principal features. First is the great beauty of the illustrations, which so far surpassed anything that had gone before that they set a new standard of excellence for all time. A very great part of the book's success is due to the superb quality of these illustrations. Second is the independence of thought which Vesalius exhibited. From his own dissections he concluded that Galen was wrong, and was describing not man but the anthropoid apes, whose anatomy he then extended to man. No longer was Vesalius correcting errors of transcription. He was correcting Galen, and claimed more than two hundred instances where the Pergamite had failed to give a true description.[28] Although others had recommended that we should rely on our own observation rather than on authority, Vesalius really carried this precept into action. He was, we might suggest, the first great modern master of the "autopsy." While this term now connotes a pathologist's examination, this is not the literal meaning. "Autopsy" means to see for one's self. Usage implicates pathology, but it should be just as applicable to normal anatomy. Vesalius looked for himself.

The matter, however, is a little more complicated. Every anatomist who dissects looks at what he is doing. Yet for the most part, before Vesalius the anatomists looked but did not see. Discrepancies between what they looked at, and what they read in Galen, simply did not "click." Awareness of contradiction was lacking. The genius is the one who first of all appreciates discrepancy, then evaluates it, and follows the path where it leads.

The *De fabrica* contains a considerable number of erroneous observations, many of which simply perpetuate the errors that Galen had already committed. Montague,[29] noting this fact, insists on Vesalius' over-all dependence on Galen. This we may freely grant. Vesalius was a Galenist who improved on his master to a profound degree, even though he himself made many erroneous and inadequate observations. Fortunately, however, progress in science does not demand perfection in each advance: it is enough that the correct road is indicated, and the early steps taken.

III

As the sixteenth century passed into the seventeenth the new concepts of science and scientific method gathered force. Reliance on experience and observation, on learning from nature, not from books, was a key point. Although we must omit the general scientific development of the period, we should at least mention Francis Bacon (1561–1626) who helped promote the new empiricism—respect for facts, but facts tempered and elaborated by judicious reasoning. Reason must be subject to facts. We should go from observation to theory, which in time should lead us to new facts. The true method of experience "first lights the candle, and then by means of the candle shows the way; commencing as it does with experience duly ordered and digested . . . and from it educing axioms, and from established axioms again new experiments."[30]

Bacon extensively discussed the proper methods of investigation. Much of what he wrote is faulty, yet much of his analysis is exceedingly keen, penetrating to the causes of error. However, we must realize that he was a theorist and philosopher, not a scientific investigator.

It is not entirely clear how much direct influence Bacon exerted on his contemporaries or immediate successors. William Harvey (1578–1657) thought that Bacon philosophized like a Lord Chancellor. Nevertheless, despite the derogatory implication, Harvey himself exemplified the scientific procedures that Bacon had so clearly enunciated. We may perhaps hold that both men drank from the same fountain of inspiration, but whereas Bacon philosophized, Harvey experimented.

Harvey, born at Folkestone and educated at Cambridge, studied medicine at Padua, where he received his doctor's degree in 1602. Returning to London as a practicing physician, he was also a member of the College of Physicians, and lectured on anatomy and physiology. Some of his manuscript notes of 1616 clearly indicate that even then he affirmed the circulation of the blood, but not until 1628 did he publish the epoch-making *De motu cordis*.[31] The details of his life, the debt he owed to his predecessors and the development of the circulation concept, are discussed in all medical history texts and innumerable journal articles, and need not be repeated here.

For the most part Harvey's methodology was implicit in his work, but he occasionally discussed certain scientific principles. He insisted on the primacy of observation. It is essential to find out whether a phenomenon does in fact happen, even if we know not how it comes about or why it occurs, and regardless whether tradition or authority are opposed.[32] In other words, *what* happens is more important that *why* or even *how* it happens.[33] Observation was more important than authority, and Harvey stressed experiment and ocular demonstration. We learn "not from books but from dissections, not from the tenets of

philosophers but from the fabric of Nature."[34] He insisted
on an appropriate relation between facts and the conclusions drawn from those facts. It is the judgment of the
senses which tests whether statements are rightly or
wrongly spoken.[35]

Harvey was a very remarkable investigator who not
only observed carefully but reasoned accurately. His inferences did not outrun the evidence but rested on a secure
base. It is important to realize that Harvey's doctrine of
the circulation represents not an observation but a chain
of reasoning based on evidence. He did not *see* the blood
go from a given point, say the right ventricle, proceed
through the lungs and back to the left heart, thence
through the rest of the body and finally return to the starting point to complete a "circle." But that the blood did
pursue this course was an inference, based on observations.
A process of reasoning "explained" or "accounted for" the
observed facts. And his concept of circulation was the only
inference that could satisfactorily explain the facts.

Harvey's evidence was abundant and quite varied. Many
individual observations, from a variety of disciplines,
dovetailed to support his conclusions. He combined comparative anatomy and embryology, *in vivo* observations of
various types and post-mortem dissections. It was not
enough, he pointed out, to dissect only dead humans, but
many different animal species, alive and dead, could furnish data for his thesis.[36]

One problem was the way in which the blood passed
from the veins and the right heart over to the left heart
and the arteries. That blood did pass was apparent. But
how? Galen had asserted that passage occurred across the
septum, through pores that were not directly observable.
Harvey denied this, and declared that all the blood passed
from the right heart to the left by traversing the lungs.

Harvey supported his contention by various observations. He analyzed the structure of the heart and great vessels, pointing out the similarities between the right and left sides, especially in regard to the valves. He argued (as had Galen in other contexts) that similarity in structure indicated similarity in function. The embryological development of the heart and evidence of comparative anatomy added further data. Fish, which lack lungs, do not have a right ventricle; and in the mammalian fetus, in which the lung does not function, the right ventricle is bypassed. It seemed clear that a right ventricle was correlated with respiration. Harvey[87] adduced a great many observations which were inconsistent with Galen's hypothesis, but the specific data and the arguments that accompanied them need not be recounted here.

Most of the facts that Harvey described were not new. But the important feature is that he emphasized the discrepancies between observed data and Galenic theory. The facts were known, but their intense relevance had hitherto been disregarded. It is only when some ignored or disregarded facts—rough edges, so to speak—become vigorously intrusive, that an explanatory theory, hitherto accepted, is critically re-examined. Why do facts, which have long been known but disregarded, one day become so intrusive and compelling? Why does a known fact suddenly become intensely relevant, even crucial and central, whereas previously it had remained peripheral and unattended? No simple answer can be given. Some individual, however, has that peculiar quality of insight which "sees" a relevance, a connection, a relation, that previously no one had noted.

"Facts" and "relationships" are quite distinct. "Discrepancy" or "inconsistency" represents a relationship whose appreciation may truly be an act of creative insight. Something "clicks" in the prepared and inquiring mind. Even though there may be cultural and educational factors which make the insight somewhat easier in one era than in another, the flash of appreciation is nevertheless the essence.

Harvey's objections to Galen were, however, a negative aspect, which required a positive or constructive aspect for completion. To prove a definite circulation Harvey advanced three propositions. "Tria confirmanda veniunt: quibus positis, necessario hanc sequi veritatem et rem palam esse, arbitror."[38] I would diverge from Franklin's translation and render this passage: "Three propositions need confirmation: if these are established, then I believe this truth [which I advocate] necessarily follows and the matter becomes plain." The three concepts are: first, that the blood is continuously transmitted by the heartbeat, "from the vena cava into the arteries in such amount that it cannot be supplied from the ingesta, and then . . . the whole mass of the blood passes across from the vena cava into the arteries within a short space of time";[39] second, that the blood is continuously driven through the arteries into every part of the body; and third, that the veins are constantly returning the blood from the periphery to the region of the heart. If these can be established, then a circulation of the blood is apparent. The demonstration of these three features beyond any reasonable doubt was brilliantly achieved, combining direct observation, mathematical calculation, conclusive experiment, straightforward and inescapable reasoning.

Everyone should read for himself this great masterpiece of scientific method. There are two aspects, however, that call for comment. Part of Harvey's general doctrine involved the claim that all the blood, impelled by the force of the right ventricle, passed through the lungs and then returned to the left side of the heart. Harvey could not demonstrate this in any direct fashion, but relied on the power of reason. He could not show how it took place, but indicated that it *must* take place, i.e., this movement was a logical necessity, and therefore true whether we could see it or not. He did not know anything about capillaries or a continuous preformed pathway. He supported his point by analogy. The blood, he thought, permeates through the lungs as water permeates through the earth's substance, or sweat passes through the skin, or urine through the kidneys, or juice of the food, carried to the liver, permeates through that organ.[40] He knew that the blood entered the lung from the right heart, and left the lung to return to the left heart. Therefore, the blood *necessarily* passed through the lung, even if the pathway was unknown. This was a requirement of reason. Only later were the pulmonary capillaries discovered, and the missing link supplied. Meanwhile it was postulated, not demonstrated.

We may point out that Galen, who ignored certain facts that Harvey stressed, nevertheless used a comparable method. If we neglect certain facts, then we might logically insist that the blood *must* pass through the cardiac septum, even though we cannot indicate just how. It was not Galen's reasoning that was incorrect but his premises, that is, his foundation of fact. Time has proved Galen wrong and Harvey right, but we must not condemn Galen's method simply because it led to a wrong conclusion.

Harvey achieved a superb blend of accurate observation and sound inference. But he too went astray when he allowed his inferences to outrun his evidence. For better understanding of subsequent theorists it is worthwhile pointing out an error, small in itself but significant from a methodological viewpoint.

Harvey discussed the passage of blood from the arteries to the veins. Ordinarily, if a suitable ligature is placed on the arm, and a vein below the ligature is opened, the blood can be drained off from the whole body. This flow of blood comes from the heart whose forceful beat drives the blood through the arteries underneath the ligature. Yet, he pointed out, under certain conditions such as fear, or "faintness," or "mental disturbance," the heart will beat more feebly and only a few drops of blood will escape from the severed vein. The reason he gave was that "the feebler heart beat and weaker driving force are unable to open the compressed artery and push the blood past the ligature, indeed, the weakened and feeble heart cannot direct the blood through the lungs or transfer it in adequate amount from the veins to the arteries." Considering that Harvey knew nothing about vasoconstriction and the mechanisms of shock, his observations were quite acute. But he went on to declare, *"In the same way and for the same reasons* the menstrual fluxes of women, and indeed all kinds of hemorrhage, subside."[41] Here, of course, he went astray. Appparently assuming that different kinds of bleeding were generically the same, he indicated that cessation of bleeding has the same cause and the same mechanism in all types of hemorrhage. Circulatory collapse or shock may bring hemorrhage to a stop, but this does not mean that the menses terminate because of circulatory collapse.

Obviously, Harvey did not know the dynamics of circulatory control, or of hormonal activity, or of hemorrhagic phenomena. Nevertheless, the knowledge he did possess would have been quite adequate to test his assertion. He needed only to perform a venesection on a woman as her period was coming to an end. The uterine bleeding would have stopped, but the blood would flow readily from the arm. This would indicate a crucial difference between the two phenomena, and that there is more than one cause for cessation of bleeding.

In this particular case Harvey committed an error against scientific method. From one phenomenon he noted certain data and drew appropriate conclusions. Then he took these data and conclusions and *applied them uncritically* to a different phenomenon, assuming that the two phenomena were similar and that what is true of the one was true of the other. Francis Bacon had already issued a warning against this error: "The best demonstration by far is experience, if it go not beyond the actual experiment. For if it be transferred to other cases which are deemed similar, unless such transfer be made by a just and orderly process, it is a fallacious thing."[42]

Error of this type, prevalent at all times, is rampant even in our enlightened mid-twentieth century. The moral is that even the best and most clear-sighted investigators are truly clear-sighted in only a circumscribed area; and for the rest they accept data or opinions more or less on faith, without critical testing. It is not enough to assert or imply similarities. It is necessary to have recourse to experience, and to see if *in fact* the similarities are demonstrable. Critical examination may disclose contradictions and inconsistencies, and thus lead to progress.

Harvey was a truly great scientist, whose great achievements were in the field of physiology rather than disease. The concept of the circulation did not by itself greatly alter his medical practice, his everyday handling of patients, his diagnosis and treatment of particular diseases. Nor did his discovery immediately change the explanations offered for disease states. However, some of the other great advances in seventeenth-century science combined to give a new viewpoint. Terrestrial and celestial mechanics analyzed the motion of bodies, large and small; the microscope disclosed very small particles within the animal body; newer anatomical studies, especially injection techniques, revealed the tremendously complex system of vessels in the body. The stage was indeed set for a new system of explanation, whereby particles in motion, obeying mechanical laws and circulating through the body, could "explain" all phases of health and disease, in accordance with the rapidly developing "mechanical philosophy."

Francis Bacon had shown the theoretical pathway. Harvey, Newton, Malpighi, Leeuwenhoek, to mention but a few, achieved great triumphs. It seemed as if all problems would yield to the new science as the age of the Enlightenment came into being.

IV

Medical theory participated in the changed attitude. As an example we may take Friedrich Hoffmann (1660–1742). Born in Halle, in Saxony, he was educated in philosophy and mathematics before studying medicine. In addition he won considerable renown as a chemist, and in his travels and further studies acquired the esteem of Robert Boyle, whom he met in London. In 1693 Hoffmann was appointed professor of medicine at the newly established University at Halle, and there earned great fame as a teacher and practitioner of medicine. He was almost sixty when he began his great work, the *Medicina rationalis systematica,* published from 1728–40.[43] His was a quiet life of academic distinction and professional accomplishment.

As we shall see, Hoffmann's career illustrates the way that raw enthusiasm can overwhelm critical judgment, another danger that Bacon pointed out. Inference can readily go awry, and lead to error rather than truth. Bacon feared that "through the premature hurry of the understanding to leap or fly to universals and principles of things, great danger may be apprehended."[44] He had criticized the "chemists" who, "out of a few experiments of the furnace have built up a fantastic philosophy, framed

159

with reference to a few things."[45] His criticism applies to Hoffmann, and, we must say with sorrow, to many twentieth-century investigators.

Apparently, however, Hoffmann had learned well the lessons which Bacon had proclaimed—the importance of proper evidence, the need for critical evaluation, the futility of purely "verbal" explanations, avoidance of dogmatism, and the necessity of sound logical inference. Hoffmann paid lip service to the scientific method. Those physicians, he declared, were truly deserving of praise "who, aspiring after truth, put aside all prejudice and are slaves to no opinion; but evaluate all things with an open mind and sound judgment; they wisely doubt mere opinions, accept nothing unless it is clear, ready, simple, and intelligible . . . deliver themselves to no sect or hypothesis totally, but rather examine all things according to the evidence and select whatever is useful and consonant to the truth, rejecting straightway those various opinions which give rise to harmful dissensions in practice and theory."[46] This constitutes a most admirable program. We can gain profound insight into the eighteenth-century mind if we study how these fine precepts worked out in practice.

An outstanding product of the Enlightenment, Hoffmann had a logical and orderly mind and a love of system. He was not nearly so rigorous as Spinoza (1632–77), who philosophized *more geometrico* and discussed the universe in definitions, axioms, and propositions which he "proved" logically. But Hoffmann did incline in that direction. He started with definitions and first principles, tried to be logical throughout, and to form a closely-knit system in which every part would have its rational explanation. Only by such sound theory, he thought, could we be sure of sound practice. The physician, he declared, should do nothing, undertake nothing, without sound reasons.[47] He must explain how diseases come about, show just how

160

various symptoms follow logically from the cause, and just how a remedy produces a cure. This is possible only if the physician thoroughly *understands* the pathogenesis.

The physician, then, cannot act scientifically or wisely unless he knows the true causes of the disease, the reasons for the symptoms, and the ways in which remedies act. He must be able to connect it all up in logical fashion. But this knowledge of causes must be of a strictly physical kind. All reasons which a physician may offer, unless based on physics or anatomy, must be considered mere speculations and creations of the mind.[48] Hoffmann objected to invoking as causes mere names which explained nothing and did not represent anything real. That is to say, all the "faculties" or "hidden powers" or "occult virtues" were completely inadmissible as causal principles. They were purely imaginary. Real causes, on the contrary, were those properties and effects which mechanical or chemical or anatomical experiment could exhibit. Physical or chemical principles founded on experiment were alone acceptable.[49]

This was a very basic premise for the physicians who adhered to the "mechanical philosophy": that there is a fundamental distinction between an imaginary force or power, and a property which could be demonstrated by experiment. The eighteenth-century rationalists, the thinkers of the Enlightenment, had great faith in the power of demonstration. It is by "just demonstration" that difficult things are made easy, the unknown made known and the obscure rendered clear. Any principle which cannot be clearly demonstrated must be rejected: "An obscure principle which can be neither defined nor conceived is unsuitable for demonstration."[50] Consequently such ancient principles as innate heat, natural moisture, crasis or dyscrasia of the humors, the faculties of the soul, the internal vital sense, the archeus of Van Helmont (or Paracelsus), were quite unacceptable. These were all merely

161

specious names, he thought, which cannot be explained and which explain nothing, which are of no value in studying the causes or effects of medical phenomena. He considered them to be merely the "recourse of lazy minds."[51]

The proper foundation for medicine was quite different. It was twofold. One aspect was *experience,* the other *reason.* "Experience" did not refer to casual or lucky observation or to chance incidents but demanded what we would call critical acumen. "True experience arises from very numerous observations, noted with great diligence, attention, and care. These embrace the entire course of the diseases and all relevant circumstances."[52] True experience we can acquire only with difficulty and with long observation, for human bodies are subject to great variations in strength, climate, season, mode of life, habits, age, temperament, and innate disposition.[53]

Experience must be supplemented by reason. From numerous particular cases we must draw general rules.[54] There must be rational explanation of effects by their causes. And from truths or principles that are well established we may, by a geometrical type of reasoning, deduce the unknown.[55] In brief, from many particulars, carefully observed, we rise to general principles. These must be related to each other in a logical manner, and then, by proper deductive reasoning, we can derive new information, hitherto unknown, from our established first principles. All this is clearly expressed or implied in Hoffmann's writings, and indicates how thoroughly he had assimilated the so-called scientific method. The Baconian seed had indeed germinated. The fruit, however, was rather disappointing.

Hoffmann was one of the great "system-makers" of the eighteenth century. Systems derive directly from the methods of science as then conceived. How reasonable it all seems: careful empirical observation will lead to generalizations which relate logically to each other and permit inference. Because our general principles and "laws" are logically intertwined, we may arrange them in a deductive order, after the model of geometry, whereby all details may ultimately derive from a few first principles. This, of course, is still the ideal of science. The eighteenth-century system-makers were not wrong in their ideals. They failed to realize, however, that ideals can never be achieved; nor did these physicians perceive how little progress they had made on their chosen path.

Hoffmann considered the two important scientific subjects on which all medicine is based to be anatomy and physics. Neglect of these was undoubtedly the cause of all the errors and dissensions of the various sects. He interpreted these basic subjects in a broad fashion. Anatomy included autopsy examinations and also the actions or, as we would say, the physiology, of the various parts.[56] Physics, which studied the movement of bodies, was the fundamental discipline. Chemistry was much less important. Hoffmann derided those writers who "explained" diseases by salts, acids, caustics, and "ferments," and ignored the mechanical properties of the bodily parts.[57] He did not entirely neglect or ignore the chemical properties of things, but relegated them, nevertheless, to a distinctly secondary position.

Hoffmann considered motion as the ruling principle for the body:

We learn by careful observation that motion is the cause of all bodily changes, that in motion also lies the basis of life and health; that the very causes of diseases act upon the solid and fluid parts of our body in no other way than through motion; nor do therapeutic agents exert their effect except by motion. Therefore, in explaining medical phenomena and therapeutic activity, we consider that special attention should be paid to motion, and to motility or the disposition of bodies [to movement], and their pathways.[58]

The body, then, is a machine put together in such a way as to produce motion. Machines are so constructed, their separate parts so interconnected, that one defective part can distort the regular movement of other parts. In a watch, for example, a fault in a single tooth in a wheel may disturb the entire machine. In similar fashion, he thought, the human body has all its parts so united and co-ordinated that disturbance of one part is communicated to all, and the normal regular movements are disturbed.[59] Hoffmann's concise summary is quite clear: "Life and death are mechanically conditioned and depend only on mechanical and physical causes which act by necessary laws."[60]

The older discussions of life and death relied on concepts such as vital action, and conjunction of soul and body. Obscure terms such as soul, spirit, archeus, or principle of life, explained nothing, offered no insight, and were of no value for making discoveries.[61] The new science, which Hoffmann represented, depended on mechanics and the principles of motion.

But motion of what? Not of any metaphysical or hypothetical substances, for these were inadmissible. Hoffmann built his system on what was clearly demonstrable. The great medical advance of the seventeenth century was the discovery of the circulation of the blood. It was the blood that moved, and it was the action of the heart which moved the blood. The ultimate cause was the movement of the finest fibers which constituted the heart and the vessels. "Motion, therefore, through which is accomplished everything that occurs in our bodies, and which the physician must use in his demonstrations, is nothing else than the contraction and expansion or, according to the Greeks,

164

the systole and diastole, of the nervous and muscular fibers and—formed from these—of the heart and arteries, and all the ducts through which all kinds of fluids circulate. . . ."[62]

Here, of course, is a mammoth *non sequitur*. Hoffmann started with observations: the blood circulates; the heart (and great vessels) contract and expand; there are many different kinds of fibers in the body. All these he could see. Then, through what he considered to be "just reasoning," he reached a conclusion which is not fact but only a faulty inference: namely, that the basic and fundamental vital process is the contraction and expansion of fibers. To understand his error, we must appreciate the limitations of his knowledge. The term "fiber" was not well defined. Microscopic studies were extremely rudimentary. The "fibers" of the eighteenth century were, very largely, the logical extrapolations of a few primitive observations. Furthermore, there was a logical need to have some elemental building-stones. Motion of the heart he could see, but the heart was not an elementary structure. It was composed of simpler parts. The fiber seemed to be the logical component. Hence he claimed that the contractile and expansile properties—i.e., the motion—of individual fibers were the elemental function. And not only of the heart, but of life generally.[63]

Hoffmann committed the *nothing but* fallacy, that besetting sin of the eighteenth-century theorists. Contraction takes place. This is true. But that *therefore everything which takes place in our body is nothing else but contraction and expansion,* is a great fallacy. Hoffmann, in maintaining this, unwittingly gave up his pretensions to sound method.

According to Hoffmann, motion is the sole cause ("causa unica") which guards all vital movements, keeps the body from putrefaction, regulates all excretions and secretions, and preserves all the functions of mind and body. Actually he was talking about circulation, which he considered the chief principle to explain bodily functions. When the circulation is free, the body is healthy. In all diseases there is some impediment to the circulation. The causes of diseases act by disturbing the vital motions, secretions, and excretions, and to achieve a cure we should "restore the free motion and circulation of the blood."[64]

It is of considerable interest to review some of Hoffmann's beliefs regarding the circulation. If the heart's motion ceases, or the movement of the blood is interrupted, then syncope or death will result. Among the causes of death he noted a wound of the heart or great vessels, through which a man bleeds to death; or, a "polypus" in the great vessels, which would kill by preventing influx of blood to the heart. ("Polypus" was the descriptive term for a post mortem clot in the heart, which was thought to be a genuine pathologic phenomenon and a frequent cause of death.) These quite obviously interrupted the circulation by mechanical means. Moreover, intense cold could kill a man, because it "coagulated" the blood.[65] This would represent a different phenomenon but still one of a mechanical character.

Just as in the body as a whole, death followed circulatory failure, so also in the parts of the body, local interruption of circulation led to corruption and local death. Tying off the vessels to a part, or very intense constriction, led to stagnation and putrefaction. Life he defined as the circulatory movement of the blood and humors, which keeps the body from corruption and regulates its functions. Plants and vegetables are not alive. To be sure, they grow and possess their own juices which move, and furthermore they wither away, yet all this is not properly regarded as life, since plants lack a heart and blood.[66]

The theoretical basis of health would appear to be quite

simple: to maintain a sound circulation. Because narrow-
ing of the vessels (as in old age) interferes with nutrition
and secretion, there result stagnations, obstructions, and
very many chronic and acute diseases. The physician must
try to keep patent the very fine vascular channels.[67] But
Hoffmann recognized, apparently, that this formulation
was not good enough, for no simple mechanical explanation would account for the facts of sepsis and "corruption."
He appreciated that very slight injuries such as the exci-
sion of corns of the foot, or a badly performed venesection,
or puncture of nerve or tendon, could lead to fatal inflammation with fever and delirium.[68] The facts of putrefaction and corruption were all too intrusive, yet their explanation was very difficult. Hoffmann recognized clinical
infection, but had no knowledge of specific agents. He
could not distinguish between bacterial infection, the necrosis from shutting off a blood supply, and post mortem
putrefaction.

To explain putrefaction Hoffmann went beyond the
purely mechanical and quantitative principles on which he
had so far placed reliance, and used a qualitative hypothetical principle. He conceived of a very subtle fluid, a
"noble," spirituous, very active substance, so extremely
tenuous that it is imperceptible and is known only by its
effects.[69] This derived quite frankly from the "spirits" of
the ancients. We recall that Galen had invoked the natural, the vital, and the animal spirits, as agents responsible
for different bodily functions. Hoffmann retained the concept of a very delicate fluid responsible for vital activity.
The great elastic power of the heart, arteries, and other
channels depended not on their own mechanical structure,
but on the subtle expansive and active fluids brought there
partly by the blood vessels, partly by the nerves. The two
elastic fluids thus brought into the heart substance caused
the contraction.[70]

Hoffmann emphasized the nervous fluid, the lineal descendent of the animal spirits. Said Hoffmann, "It is not the mind, nor the sensitive soul which is the adequate, constant, and proximal cause of the vital motions of systole and diastole, by which all natural actions take place. But it is a very delicate fluid, warm, elastic, contained in the finest tubules of the membranes and nerves and in the blood itself, which is the cause of these motions, and of life, health, and diseases."[71] Needless to say, he did not demonstrate this fluid. He merely hypothesized that it existed.

When he used concepts such as these, Hoffmann diverged from his avowed mechanical principles. Thus, he believed that diastole and systole were separate movements, each with its own cause. The blood within the vessels produced diastole by its abundance and its expansive heat. This, of course, would represent a mechanical activity. Then he claimed that the active fluid which passed into the heart through the nerves and coronary vessels caused the succeeding contraction. But this would be a "vital stimulation," and to say that it is mechanical merely begs the question. To assert that a hypothetical fluid acts mechanically, when neither the fluid nor its action is demonstrated, is a serious breach of logic.

An imperceptible substance may indeed exist. If we cannot detect it directly through the senses, we may recognize its effects and infer that *something* is acting to produce the phenomena. But how can we assume that this *something*, whatever it is, whose existence is known only through its effects, is a material entity which obeys the laws of mechanics and exerts its effect through the principles of mechanical motion? This is sheer gratuitous assumption and blandly assumes what needs to be proven. The vital activity we observe. The explanation of that activity we merely infer. There is no more warrant for declaring that the cause is a material substance which obeys mechanical principles than there is for asserting that an archeus, or a ferment, or a "vital principle" is responsible. Hoffmann, of course, is relying on faith, not on direct evidence. Classical mechanics, that is, the laws governing bodies in motion, can explain some bodily phenomena. Therefore he assumed these laws can explain all bodily phenomena.

Hoffmann obviously could not define this subtle fluid representing the vital principle. Nevertheless, he believed that whatever it is which nourishes, invigorates, and animates us, which moves the blood and bestows strength on body and mind, is of a material nature and exists in the blood.[72] He declared, "The blood is therefore most properly called the treasury of life, the vehicle of the vital principle and the link between this and the body."[73] The blood, he thought, was a mixture of many different parts, solid and fluid, heavy and light, transparent and fixed, watery and earthy. It contained an inflammable oil.[74] Four ounces of blood, if heated, will yield up one ounce of solid material. Therefore, he believed, we should ingest three times as much fluids as solids, in order that the blood should maintain the proper ratio of liquids to solids.

Hoffmann recognized the great complexity of the blood. His analytical techniques were very primitive, heat and distillation playing a major role, but he also utilized direct naked eye observation and some elemental microscopy. Moreover he relied heavily on analogies. For example, he noted many points of resemblance between blood and gelatine. Both are easily hardened by cold. When the watery parts evaporate they both become a "gluten." Acids induce coagulation in both. Since blood has a "gelatinous nature," it follows, he declared, that foods which give a gelatinous juice when cooked, or contain a gelatinous principle, are most suitable for forming good blood. Animal foods—meats—thus are most effective in blood regeneration following blood loss. Foods in which saline, acid,

169

spirituous, or earthy substances predominate are less effective in increasing the blood.[75] It is interesting to note, in passing, how similar are these ideas to the work of Whipple and Robscheit-Robbins[76] over two hundred years later.

There were, of course, distinctions between blood and gelatine. Distillation indicated quantitative differences in the relative proportions of volatile salts and oils. Furthermore, blood became far more putrid, producing a much greater stench than did gelatine. In fact, no other substance became as putrid and corrupt as did human blood. Hoffmann concluded that blood could be considered a refined and subtle gelatine.[77] Considering the crude modes of discrimination then available, this was a significant contribution to protein chemistry.

However, he ran into great difficulties through his uncritical analogies. A few observations he puffed up into a mammoth but very insubstantial structure. Where he lacked positive knowledge about details, he often filled the gap with what he considered to be logical inferences. But whereas logic may sometimes anticipate observation, it cannot replace it. In other words a theory must eventually somehow be verified through perceptual experience if it is to hold up. Hoffmann all too frequently neglected this, and his doctrines suffered correspondingly. For example, he tried to explain fever by combining certain data of heat and of motion, and declared that the heat of the blood depends almost entirely on the violent motion of its "subtle sulfurous parts." As these sulfurous parts increase, or their agitation intensifies, the total motion is increased. Therefore, according to this line of reasoning, the more rapid the circulation, as in fever or exercise, the more intense the heat.[78] Thus he "explains" fever on mechanical grounds.

The complexity of the blood was an ever-intrusive fact. He believed that the blood contains elements of diverse

nature and properties, but that the internal motion mixes
and unites these to produce a homogeneous vital fluid.
Blood placed in a glass tube and examined microscopically
appeared like water in which were innumerable reddish
globules, "which are nothing else than the gelatinous and
sulfurous part of the blood which, divided by the motion
and inward agitation, assumes a globose configuration. All
heterogeneous [particles] shaken up in a different fluid,
assume a globose configuration, and the more these globules are divided, to become smaller and more numerous,
to that extent the blood is more fluid, more florid, and
more appropriate for safeguarding the vital circulation:
but in proportion as the globules are fewer and larger, to
that extent the blood is thicker and darker."[79]

Hoffmann was indeed an early hematologist, who made
a plea for hematology as an important discipline. He
appreciated the variations in blood in respect to consistency, color, and "power" ("virtus"). These differences he
accounted for through numerous variables such as the food
ingested, disposition of the vessels, structure of the solids,
or the patient's race, temperament, habitus, modes of exercise, or blood-letting regimen. All these may affect the appearance of the blood.[80] Moreover, the appearance varied
in health and disease. Therefore he urged the physician to
learn the different characteristics of the blood. He recommended taking the specific gravity. The vital fluid should
be not too thick and black, nor too thin and red, but should
be in a mean proportion. If the blood is so thick that the
serum becomes a lard-like gluten, this suggests a severe inflammation or a chronic disease. Serum that is too abundant indicates a weakness in secretion of liver and kidneys,
and such diseases as scabies, arthritis, and scurvy (which
all arise from an "impure serum"). Blood which is too
fluid and dark red, and does not coagulate, is very bad. This

is seen in patients who die of plague, hectic fever, consumption, pox, and acute fevers.[81]

It is not our purpose to cover, in this volume, the many physiological and pathological states that Hoffmann described. His general method and certain of his presuppositions have already been indicated. Of particular interest is the interconnection of bodily parts and functions that played such a significant role in this system. The body was indeed a machine, but one whose fluid and solid parts influenced each other in remarkable fashion. Disturbance in one part is widely communicated to other parts. This he called "consensio," which is best translated as "sympathy," in the special sense of accord between different areas. By this concept he "explained," in purely verbal fashion, many different disease conditions. Disturbance of the heartbeat can affect the mind and the state of consciousness; activity of hands or feet can affect the entire circulation. A small amount of blood remaining immovable in very small vessels—Hoffmann's formulation for inflammation—may cause the entire body to suffer, so that there is not only local pain, redness, and swelling, but fever and thirst as well. That is, systemic symptoms may result from local inflammation. All of these indicate "sympathy."[82] The nerves, he realized, played a very important part in this communication. Anticipating Broussais, he emphasized that the stomach and intestines show especially rich connections with other bodily functions. A small erosion of the stomach can produce vomiting, convulsions, cold sweat, and not infrequently a fatal outcome (presumably indicating death from peritonitis). In infants the mere distention of the gums by erupting teeth may be fatal, with fevers, delirium, and convulsions. And very minor operations may induce disastrous inflammation.[83]

There was a "consent" between the blood circulating in the vessels and the subtle fluids in the nerves. When the blood stagnates in vessels, Hoffmann believed that the nerves were abnormally affected, and thrown into a spasm. Pain, fever, hemorrhage, and suppression of excretions may result. From too great distention, or from erosion of the nervous elements, the pulse is altered, the vessels constricted, and blood flow impaired.[84]

This emphasis on "sympathies," whether through the nerves or the circulation, indicates an important methodological point. Hoffmann gave many examples where rather minor disturbances were followed by profound reactions. There seemed to be a marked disproportion between the trivial cause and the severe effect. We today would say that some additional causal factors were operative, factors which, if not known, must be postulated in order to achieve a due proportionality between cause and effect. Hoffmann, however, did not reason in this way and bridged the gap with a word. A trivial cause, of itself insignificant, becomes significant through the operation of "sympathy" or "consent." This is saying, in essence, that a small cause spreads, and merely by its spread produces a large effect. He did not perceive that a grave logical hiatus existed.

Judged by later standards, Hoffmann exhibited much confusion. He mixed up many different biological processes which today we can discriminate. Although he noted many observational sequences, he could not perceive the intermediate steps between the terms of these sequences. He nevertheless tried to connect them through his own vague terminology, largely borrowed. The vital principles, the subtle fluids, the lively stimulating qualities, the sympathies and consents—these were connecting links with which he tied together various data. The observations were often quite accurate, but his explanatory concepts were not adequate.

Hoffmann was indeed rather hobbled by his too great

dependence on the mechanical philosophy. Nature appeared relatively simple. Particles in motion according to the laws of mechanics, too much or too little blood, channels too wide or too narrow, these seemed quite adequate explanations. To be sure, it was also necessary to invoke various "subtle" factors, which meant, in essence, that nobody knew much about them. And, as we have noted, to assert that "subtle" factors were mechanical was merely begging the question. There were a lot of observations which could not be smoothly fitted into the mechanical philosophy. Instead of discarding this philosophy, Hoffmann chose to squeeze the data until they superficially harmonized with avowed principles. Further progress developed only after the "subtle" factors were carefully analyzed, and when the previous observations were reexamined. New techniques, new tools, played a tremendous role in permitting a fruitful re-examination.

Cell Theory, Key to
Modern Medicine

BOERHAAVE, SCHWANN, ROKITANSKY,
VIRCHOW

Starting in the later eighteenth century, and developing with great rapidity in the nineteenth century, medical theory and practice began a massive upsurge, just as if a seed had finished a long germination and then sprouted with startling vigor. There were tremendous advances in the basic sciences, especially in chemistry and physiology, and in the fields of clinical observation as well. At the same time there developed a new awareness of critical standards, of which statistical analysis is merely one facet. New observations and new theoretical advances transformed medical thinking and extended medical horizons far beyond what Hoffmann could have imagined. One of the great seminal concepts of the nineteenth century was the so-called "cell theory," by which we mean that the units of biological structure are microscopic bodies called cells, with certain definable characters.

It was Robert Hooke who applied the term "cell" to biology. In 1664, describing the structure of petrified wood, he noted the conspicuous "pores" identical with the "microscopical pores" of wood. In 1665 he mentioned the similar closely-set pores in charcoal, and especially described the texture of cork, which was perforated with spaces not unlike a honeycomb. These spaces he called "pores, or cells."[1] Reproductions of his original illustration and a picture of the microscope he used are to be found, for example, in Wolf[2] or Hughes.[3]

The term "cell" found ready acceptance, but originally signified a space, surrounded by a boundary wall. When transferred to animal tissues, it had a sense entirely different from its modern significance. In the seventeenth and eighteenth centuries "cellular tissue" was a term essentially of gross description. It referred to the loose connective (or "areolar") tissue of the body, where fibrous strands bounded actual or potential spaces. This loose cellular tissue could, for example, be readily distended by air. Or, fluid under pressure could infiltrate the spaces, separate the boundary fibers, and "fill" the "cells." Hence, when, in the eighteenth century we encounter the words "cell" and "cellular," we must realize that their meanings are very different from those of nineteenth-century cell theory.

Biologists and historians have studied in great detail the growth of cell theory in its anatomical or morphological aspects,[4] but less attention has been paid to the functional precursors of the cell concept. Cells represent not only structural units, elemental building-blocks which exist in great variety, but also functional units. That is, a cell is the demonstrable locus wherein a specific function is performed. Specificity of function has always been puzzling. How does it happen that the kidney secretes urine and the liver secretes bile? Why does not the liver once in a while eliminate urine? This is a very significant question, and through the ages many different answers have been suggested. Of course we could say that the liver has the "faculty" of secreting bile, a type of explanation that we have discussed previously. But such a diffuse explanation is no longer satisfactory.

Instead of pointing to the liver as a whole, we now can be more precise and point to an individual liver cell, a microscopic unit which secretes bile. But this is scarcely a proper solution. It is quite obvious if we point to a single liver cell instead of the whole liver, we only push the ultimate solution a few stages further back, since we still face the problem: How does the individual liver cell produce bile? Recent progress in intracellular chemistry has considerably advanced our knowledge, and we can speak with some assurance about a few of the mechanisms involved.

From the historical aspect we may approach cell theory through study of secretory functions. Bile, urine, milk, and sweat, for example are all different, all qualitatively specific. How to account for this difference? In the eighteenth century, long before the cell as an anatomic unit was discovered, there were many explanations and ingenious hypotheses to explain the specificity of function. Let us analyze in detail one of these hypotheses, which may be construed as a precursor of cell theory.

II

Hermann Boerhaave (1668–1738) was the leading physician in the first half of the eighteenth century. A recognized authority in chemistry and in botany, a sound mathematician, and the outstanding clinician of his era, he synthesized in his own person all the major trends in medical science. He tried to unify medical knowledge, and account for all phenomena through a few simple concepts. All these concepts, however fanciful they may seem to us today, were nevertheless ultimately founded on observation and experiment. The works of Newton, Harvey, Malpighi, Hooke, Ruysch, and other seventeenth-century writers, furnished the factual data which Boerhaave elaborated.

Boerhaave relied on certain general principles applicable to all secretions, namely, the laws of hydrodynamics which govern the motion of discrete particles in a fluid medium. In addition he maintained two basic and interlocking accessory principles: (1) that in the circulating blood there were particles of many different sizes, so different as to constitute different orders of magnitude; (2) that corresponding to different particles there were orders of vessels, of appropriately different size and arrangement.[5] Out of all this he established a system that "explained" all functions that we today attribute to cells.

That the blood contained globules was known to Swammerdam and Malpighi, but of the early writers it was Leeuwenhoek who perhaps defined them most clearly, and indicated the characteristics of the red cells. Boerhaave relied very largely on Leeuwenhoek's findings and interpretations, and unfortunately, on his errors as well. The basic observation was simple: a small amount of blood was drawn into a capillary tube, and, to facilitate examination, diluted with a little water. Then the contents were examined under a microscope. The red globules were clearly visible, but even under observation were seen to lose their color, and to break up into smaller yellowish "serous" globules. Soon, under the observer's very eyes, these particles disintegrated into still smaller elements and the eye was incapable of following the disintegration any further. This describes quite well the phenomenon we call hemolysis, but Boerhaave, following Leeuwenhoek, interpreted it differently. Obsessed by the number six, he thought that the red cells were *composed of* six smaller serous globules and each of these, in turn, was composed of six small spherules. He thought he observed the break-up of one red cell into thirty-six smaller fragments. Then, he went on, "the eye is incapable of descending any farther into smaller divisions of these last globules, but by reason and analogy we have some foundation to believe that the more subtle juices in the human body are composed of still smaller globules, and that there are as many series of decreasing globules as there are of the smaller vessels conveying the several juices."[6]

Here we have erroneous observations misinterpreted and then elaborated by "reason and analogy." This fallacious mixture served as the basis for a massive theoretical superstructure. Fundamental in this elaboration was the faith that when the red cell disintegrated, the process which we see could be extrapolated far beyond the limits of direct observation. These further subdivisions of the red cell, admittedly inferential, were nevertheless deemed rational and logical, and, in a metaphorical sense, clearly visible to the eye of reason.

Correlative with the particles were the vessels. Here again, direct observation could carry us a certain distance, and then "rational" extrapolation took us a lot further. It was very clear that there were different "orders" of vessels. The arterio-venous pathway was well defined. Harvey's discovery of the circulation had indicated a continuous preformed pathway, from large arteries to small arteries, from small arteries to those still smaller, from these to capillaries, and thence back to veins of increasing size until the largest veins of all conducted the blood back into the heart, to complete the circulation. Concerning this pathway there was no doubt. Boerhaave called this system of vessels "sanguiferous," that is, carrying the red cells.

But observation readily showed certain vessels which normally did not admit red cells. The white of the eye, for example, ordinarily showed no vessels, yet vessels of some sort were there. They were visible as angry red streaks if the eye became inflamed, and, moreover, could be rendered visible by suitable injection techniques.[7] Boerhaave's interpretation was as follows. These vessels of the eye were normally *too small* to admit red cells, and therefore *must have a diameter less than that of a red cell.* These vessels would normally admit particles *smaller* than the red cells —namely, the "yellow serous globules." Thus, he thought that there existed one series of vessels for the red globules, and a different series for the small yellow or serous globules. In disease states such as inflammation these "serous vessels" could, as part of the disease process, be filled with red globules, that is, with particles of the next larger order. But this was a pathologic phenomenon only and did not occur in physiological states.

Observations in the seventeenth century had disclosed another series of vessels, namely, the lymphatics and the lacteals, which were quite separable from the channels that carried blood. This lymphatic system, which emptied into the thoracic duct and thence into the subclavian vein, Boerhaave incorporated into his anatomical hierarchy. The red globules circulated in the sanguiferous vessels; the smaller "serous" globules in the smaller "serous" vessels; and the still smaller globules, which he called "lymphatic," circulated in the lymphatic channels. And then Boerhaave extrapolated:

Hence then, the sanguiferous arteries will carry all parts of the blood, the serous arteries will convey all but the red globules, and the lymphatics all but the red and yellow globules, etc. *and thus probably is the succession of vessels and humors continued,* till the ultimate or last series of the smallest vessels convey only the most subtle juices in the body. . . . Since therefore we are thus convinced that there are liquors in the body more subtle than the lymph, *we may rest equally satisfied that there are also smaller arteries which convey them,* and which arise from the lymphatic arteries in the same manner as they from the serous, and the serous from the sanguiferous.[8]

It is important to note how easily Boerhaave brought in his assumptions which he considered to be logical, thoroughly justifiable inferences.

The hierarchy was constructed as follows: the sanguiferous vessels, just before they open into the corresponding veins, "send off lesser arteries from their sides, which receive the yellow serum." These, in turn, before they become veins, send off the lymphatic vessels as lateral branches, "and those lymphatic arteries will detach a third series still less, and so on with the several smaller series, till they terminate in the ultimate or very smallest series of vessels in the whole body called nerves."[9] It is no part of our purpose to consider his concepts of nerve fluid.

Boerhaave's physiology depended on varying sized particles in the blood, and vessels of different sizes to accommodate them. He explained secretions in the following fashion:

He began with the food, transformed into chyle, which was "prepared in the mouth, digested in the stomach, elaborated in the intestines, secerned in the lacteals, attenuated at the mesenteric glands, and farther diluted and mix'd in the thoracic duct, then blended with the venal blood."[10] There is mixture in the right heart, and then the mixture is propelled into the lungs. Boerhaave did not accept our modern concepts regarding the functions of the lungs. He carefully examined and then rejected the theory that the lungs serve to absorb air into the blood,[11] but his analysis, fascinating as it is, is not germane to our immediate problem. For him the lungs served to convert the chyle "into nutritious juices."[12] This takes place through mechanical and hydrodynamic principles. Thus, the chyle flowing through the pulmonary vessels is subjected to special forces and pressures through the expansion and contraction of the organs, through inspirations and expirations. This activity, as the particles traverse the various series of pulmonary vessels, produce "a great attrition," whereby the particles "are broke, polished, and rounded; a compressure, by which they are densified and formed into spherules; a lubricity and aptitude for motion, by being strained through the smallest vessels of this organ."[13] The lungs in fact are the organ by which the chyle is rendered part of the blood.

The significant feature of Boerhaave's theory, however, is not the blunder, *but the role which he assigns to the vessels.* It is not the lungs per se which bring about the transformation, but the vessels in the lung which *cause the transformation of one substance into another.* Boerhaave considered that this transformation took place through mechanical forces—attrition, compression, and abrasion and the like, occurring in a fluid medium. The respiratory movement aided these mechanical processes.

It was not merely the pulmonary vessels which behaved in this fashion, but all vessels, all over the body, which *acted on* their contained material. "Acted on" is a very broad term which covers a multitude of functions, including those which we today attribute to the various chemical transformations occurring inside the cells.

Boerhaave tried to describe the action of the arteries in mechanical terms. In the arteries the particles undergo "motion, collision, and rotation . . . attrition, attenuation, and compactness . . . levigation of their angles, and an uniformity or similitude of each particle . . . with that division of its parts fitting them to pass through all the small vessels."[14] By the various abrasions and compactions, the particles of chyle and milk are converted into blood.

Furthermore, the bodily heat, which we correlate with metabolism, Boerhaave associated with the frictional heat of the blood particles, especially the red globules. The heat of the blood was deemed proportional to the velocity and number of these globules,[15] and Boerhaave showed considerable ingenuity in connecting this concept with various disease states.

With these general principles in mind, we may now consider the problems of secretion. Glands according to Boerhaave, who followed the data of Ruysch,[16] were composed of congeries of vessels. The injection studies of Ruysch had exhibited most admirably the astounding variety of the vascular pattern, their modes of branching and anastomoses. These variations, thought Boerhaave, subjected the particles to different mechanical stresses: contacts, agitations, repulsions, compressions, and attenuations.[17]

The various secretions or humors—the sweat, tears, earwax, sebaceous material, mucus, saliva, bile, milk, semen—owe their specificity to the various mechanical factors involving the small branches of the vascular system. Thus, for any secreting gland the distance from the heart, the vascular configuration, the number and arrangement of the vascular branches and their relation to the parent trunk, the propelling forces, were all considered supremely important. The blood did not contain the various humors as such, but only the formative particles which were brought to the glands and then separated. He gave the example of semen, which he deemed a secretion, and which "is secerned thin and limpid from pellucid arteries which do not admit the cruor."[18] That is, particles smaller than the red cells were separated out by vessels which were too small to receive the red globules. The separation was accomplished by mechanical forces.

Boerhaave expressly rejected the simple "pore" theory of early mechanistic doctrine. Instead he fell back on peculiarities of the vessels, of which he assumed many different orders and types. He believed that "The secretions depend very much on the fabric of the solid parts; and that the different structure of the glands in the several parts of the body will occasion different juices to be separated." The glands transmute the secreted juices "as the same juice of the earth is diversified by different plants into various liquors, so different from each other, as the bitter aloe . . . and the sweet sugar-cane." And then, as a crowning summary, he went on, "All which variety of secerned juices result from the inscrutable mechanism of the animal vessels or the vegetable tubes, the different velocity with which they are propelled, and the various combinations of their particles, etc."[19]

And yet he had his misgivings, for he went on to say, "We are therefore not yet clear in the business of all the glands and their secretions; and there are probably many artifices concealed from us in this branch of nature, which we have not so much as suspected or thought of."[20]

In summary, then, of Boerhaave's concepts, we suggest the following interpretation. Boerhaave used the term "vessel" in at least two different senses. The vessel could serve as the locus of transport from one place to another. But, in addition, some vessels were considered to be the locus of many bodily changes, such as the breakdown of complex material into simpler particles, and conversely the synthesis of complex substances from simpler ones. So too a vessel was the locus for bodily heat and all the properties we attribute to "metabolism." The ordinary blood channels visible in dissection did not seem adequate to achieve

184

all this complexity, so Boerhaave *hypothesized a whole series of invisible vessels, perceptible to the eye of reason, to account for the various metabolic functions.* He confused the visible and invisible vessels, mistakenly thinking that all the bodily functions operated on simple mechanical principles, according to movement of particles within tubes. But the tubes, both visible and hypothetical, were not inert; they "acted" on their contents, somehow, and some of his vessels correspond with the elements that later were called cells.

He suspected that all this was far short of the truth, and his poignant remark, that there is probably much that we have not yet suspected, was truly prophetic. His prophecy was fulfilled by the discovery of cells, in the modern sense.

III

The hundred years following the death of Boerhaave saw tremendous medical advances. I will mention only two. First, there was a growing emphasis on body tissues (or "textures," to use contemporary language), rather than organs; and second, an emphasis on minute observation. By this I mean concern less with broad shallow generalization and more with fine details. This took place in both clinic and laboratory, and underlay the discovery of cell theory in its modern form. Of the many individuals who contributed to the discovery of cells, it is, perhaps, Theodor Schwann (1810–82) who deserves especial credit. To celebrate the 150th anniversary of his birth, two excellent biographical and critical studies, by Florkin[21] and Watermann,[22] have recently appeared.

Schwann was born in Neuss on the Rhine, a few miles from Cologne. After receiving excellent training in mathematics and physics, he began in 1829 to study medicine at Bonn. Here the great attraction was Johannes Mueller

(1801–58) who taught comparative anatomy, physiology, and general pathology, and was one of the great seminal forces in nineteenth-century medical research. In 1834 Schwann received his M.D. from Berlin, having written his doctoral thesis on the need for atmospheric air in the development of the incubated egg ("De necessitate aeris atmospherici ad evolutionem pulli in ovo incubito").

The next few years truly revealed his investigative genius. He performed basic work on muscular contraction; he studied the proteolytic action of gastric juice, clearly defined the specific ferment pepsin and its role in the digestion of protein, and was able to isolate the enzyme in solution; he studied alcoholic fermentation and its relation to yeasts as living microorganisms, and the means whereby this activity could be inhibited; and he showed that putrefaction as well as fermentation resulted from the intervention of microorganisms. And then he first communicated his researches on cell theory, publishing in 1839 the book[23] which became one of the classics of medicine.

The early history of microscopic observations has been excellently covered in the references cited.[24] Early in the nineteenth century, it was appreciated that plant cells were more than mere spaces bounded by walls, and by the 1830's there was much productive activity among microscopists. In 1833 Robert Brown (1773–1858, the discoverer of "Brownian movement") noted the cell nucleus, or "areola," and "may be said to have established the concept of the nucleated cell as the unit of structure in plants."[25]

In his study of cells Schwann furnished the catalyzing insight which unified a great many separate observations and indicated their over-all relationships. Schleiden (1804–81), who had reported certain structural and developmental details of plant cells,[26] one day at dinner indicated to Schwann the important role that the nucleus played in cell development. Schwann recalled that certain animal structures, in cartilage and notochord, closely resembled plant cells, and he wondered whether the nuclei had the same role in the animal tissues as in vegetable cells.[27] While Valentine in 1836 and Henle in 1837 had already suggested certain similarities between plant and animal cells,[28] it was Schwann who systematically established the thesis.

In a series of brilliant researches he indicated the similarity of plant and animal cells; showed that all animal cells, despite their apparent diversity, were basically similar; and propounded a theory on structure and development of cells in the animal economy. Schwann amassed a great deal of concrete data, from which he drew logical inferences and built up a reasonable and coherent theory. Most of what both Schleiden and Schwann actually said was quite wrong; the data were incorrect and the inferences, while logical, were false. Yet his fundamental insight was valid. That the details were wrong is not so very important.

In the 1830's the microscope was still a very imperfect instrument. Techniques for preparing specimens were rudimentary. Plant material, with its relatively rigid walls, lent itself to freehand sectioning, but with softer material only spreads and squash preparations were available. Modern routine procedures, fixation, embedding, accurate sectioning, and differential staining, were not then known. Investigators sometimes used a few simple coloring agents such as iodine, or made observations after applying acetic acid, but studies were generally made on unfixed and unstained material. The available microscope lenses left much to be desired, and although considerable correction had been achieved, resolving power was low. The microscopes that Schwann, Henle, and Mueller employed could resolve points that were just under one micron apart, whereas today an ordinary student microscope, with a high dry lens, can resolve points separated by only a third of this distance,[29] and oil immersion lenses can, of course, do considerably better.

Observing fresh material in spread or squash preparations without differential staining, through microscope lenses of low resolution, was not easy. Schwann realized the difficulty of making reliable observations, and noted on occasions that what he saw was "probably an optical deception."[30] The delicate nature of the cell membrane, the similar refractive index of cell wall and cell contents, and the granular appearance which both might manifest, all intensified the difficulty. The great variety of cell forms also raised problems in recognition and identification.[31] Furthermore, the use of water as the medium for examining fresh specimens induced cellular changes which complicated any interpretation. It is not surprising that Schwann made errors. What is surprising is that he discovered so much.

Schleiden's concepts formed the basis of Schwann's doctrines. The botanist was concerned with the way that plant cells developed. The existence in cells of a special spot called the areola or nucleus was already known, and Schleiden, believing that it bore a special relation to cell development,[32] called it the cytoblast. He noted a special structure within the nucleus. In favorable specimens it was "a small, sharply defined body, which, judging from the shadow it casts, appears to represent a thick ring, or a thick-walled hollow globule." Sometimes "it appears only as a sharply circumscribed spot."[33] He believed that these small bodies (corresponding to the nucleolus) preceded the formation of the nucleus.

Schleiden studied cell formation in the early embryo sac, where, as Hughes points out,[34] the newly-formed cells do not lay down rigid cell walls. Within a "gum"-like fluid, there appeared "a quantity of exceedingly minute

granules . . . most of which, on account of their minute-
ness, look like mere black points."³⁵ Studying the relation
of granules and cells he concluded that of the many granules (nucleoli) within the plant juice, some became larger
and more sharply defined and transformed into the "cyto-
blasts" (nuclei). These, with their "granulous coagula-
tions," were at first free-lying, but when they "have attained their full size, a delicate transparent vesicle rises
upon their surface. This is the young cell, which at first
represents a very flat segment of a sphere," the flat side
formed by the cytoblast, on which the convex side rises up
"somewhat like a watch glass upon a watch."³⁶ The space
so formed is filled with fluid. The young cell expands (just
as if the watch glass grew into a total sphere, while the
watch remained the same size and in contact with the
glass). His illustrations indicate how the cell wall becomes
more and more prominent, while the nucleus may become
enclosed within the cell wall, or even absorbed.

In this analysis the significant features are, first, the
existence of granules, then the "growth" of certain particular granules into an organized structure which is the
"cytoblast." This cytoblast "produces" the cell, by somehow inducing the appearance of a surrounding structure
which grows and ultimately exhibits a firm cell wall.

In animals certain cartilagenous structures suggest a
similarity to plant tissues. Schwann had the insight that
plants and animals both developed from comparable units
or cells. If in plants the cell wall was so significant and the
nucleus so dominant, the same features should occur in
animals. If the nucleus was the "cytoblast" in plants, and
the nucleus developed from granules, the same sequence
should apply to animals. Schwann searched for granules
and nuclei, for cells and their "walls," and found them in
cartilage and notochord. But while cartilage provided a

ready comparison with plant cells, Schwann generalized the schema for all animal tissue.

There were, according to his views, two major principles: a matrix, out of which the cells arise; and the cytoblast, a formative agency or active force.

The following admits of universal application to the formation of cells; there is, in the first instance, a structureless substance present, which is sometimes quite fluid, at others more or less gelatinous. This substance [the blastema] possesses within itself, in a greater or lesser measure according to its chemical qualities and the degree of its vitality, a capacity to occasion the production of cells. When this takes place the nucleus usually appears to be formed first, and then the cell around it. The formation of cells bears the same relation to organic nature that crystallization does to inorganic."[37]

Schwann, having arrived at his concepts through studying cartilage and notochord, applied the principles to all animal tissues. These he classified into five groups. In the first category he placed the "isolated independent cells" that are found in fluids such as blood or lymph, pus or mucus, all of which contained "corpuscles," or globules enclosing a nucleus. Schwann assumed that all these cells *arose out of the fluid in which they were found,* so that the fluid portions of the pus or blood, lymph or mucus, were the "blastema" or matrix in which the cells would have the developmental course already described.

Much of what Schwann said was dictated by theoretical requirements rather than direct observations. Thus, regarding the actual formation of the pus cells, he declared in reserved fashion that it was "most likely that the nuclei of pus cells are their first formed part, but I have no investigations on the subject."[38] That is, the theory originally devised to explain one set of observations he applied *in toto* to a different area, and assumed that the theory would fit, even without positive direct evidence. At least there was as yet no evidence to the contrary, so that for a while his assumption was unchallenged.

After considering the cells which float free in the body fluids, Schwann analyzed the solid elements, which he divided into four groups. First were the epithelial tissues, wherein the individual cells, instead of lying free, were firmly applied to each other to form a coherent layer or mass. Because of technical problems he investigated principally the epithelial derivatives such as the nails, the hooves, the crystalline lens, and feathers. He found that these, in their growth, conformed to his concept of cells.

In the next category he placed those hard tissues which had a common feature, namely, that their cell walls coalesced with each other or with the intercellular substance to produce a very resistant substance. As examples he gave cartilage, bone, and the "ivory" of the teeth. In all these the constituent cells seemed to exhibit similarities to plant cells whose firm walls crowd together to give a rigid structure.

Next came the tissues whose cells convert into fibers, as are found, for example, in the connective tissues. The fibrous character of many body tissues had long been known, and the theoretical and practical importance of fibers in physiology and pathology can scarcely be overestimated.[39] To Schwann the various fibers which we would call collagen or reticulum represented an elongation of cell bodies, which later split up into the fibrillar elements. There are fibrous tissues of varying degrees of density, from the very loose to the very compact. All these he considered to be transformed cells, that is, elements which started as cells in a fashion similar to other tissues, but which underwent an elongation and then a fission. This over-all general category included the "areolar," the "fibrous," and the "elastic" tissues.

The final group included those cells whose walls coalesce and whose cell cavities communicate with each other to form continuous hollow tubes. The prime example here is a capillary network. Schwann made observations on the tail of the tadpole, but he misinterpreted his findings. There was first of all the assumption that cells were hollow. Capillaries, he thought, developed from individual cells, originally separate, of round or stellate configuration, whose processes joined one with another. Where they came in contact the cell walls became absorbed so that the cell cavities could also communicate. In this way anastomoses were formed. The original elements, before their union, he called primary cells. After fusion there was a "secondary" cell, whose cavity "consists of the united cavities of the original cells, and its cell-membrane of all their blended cell-membranes."[40] Schwann attributed this same histogenesis to muscle and nerve as well as capillaries.

While this classification seems very strange to us, founded as it is on erroneous concepts and faulty observations, we must not forget its original context. Schwann's major interest was to establish a general biological law, namely, "that there is one universal principle of development for the elementary parts of organisms, however different, and that this principle is the formation of cells."[41] The cells all originate in comparable fashion and then become transformed into the elemental components of the different tissues. To establish this thesis he investigated many different tissues. He tried to define wherein the differences lay. Correlatively, he sought common factors which applied to all types of cells, however diverse their location, arrangement, or physiological function.

The common factors were in essence two, first the growth sequence which began with a nucleolus and continued to the fully formed cell with its cell wall; and second, the matrix or mother-substance or cytoblastema, out of which the cells develop. When Schwann studied the many body tissues, all observations somehow had to harmonize with these basic concepts. Frequently there were discordant notes, and it is instructive to see how he resolved the difficulties.

The concept of cytoblastema led to many complications. How did it happen that in some fluids there were very abundant cells, in others only a few? If we regard pus, for example, we note that sometimes it is thin, bloody, with relatively few cells; at other times thick, creamy, with enormous numbers of cells in a very small fluid volume. Of this type is the so-called "healthy pus," more widely known, perhaps, as "laudable pus" (i.e., caused by a bacterium of low virulence, readily overcome by the body's defenses). Pus of this nature was a sign that the lesion would soon be cured.

Why did the "healthy pus" have more cells than an "unhealthy" type? Schwann had an answer: all cytoblastema had a "plastic force," i.e., ability to produce cells. "The more healthy the pus, the greater is its *plastic force,* and the greater the number of cells which are formed in it, so that in healthy pus the quantity of serum is very small in comparison with the number of cells."[42] Conversely, if there were only a few cells, the blastema would have had but a weak plastic force.

This, of course, is non-informative juggling with words. A "plastic force" is a "faculty" in disguise, merely rephrasing the phenomenon it purports to explain. Schwann's theories did not give any real clue to the phenomenon, but merely asserted the fact that sometimes there were a lot of cells relative to a very small amount of fluid.

What was the relation of blastema to the blood vessels? Schwann fully appreciated that cell growth required nutritive fluids which could come only from the blood. Some body components, such as ordinary connective tissue or muscle, had blood vessels more or less uniformly distributed. These tissues he called "organized." On the other hand there were tissues such as cartilage or epidermis that contained no blood vessels, and these he called "unorganized." How did these tissues grow? How did their component cells multiply and develop, in the absence of blood vessels?

Where there are no blood vessels, as in the epidermis or in cartilage, the young cells are formed "only in the neighborhood of that surface, on which they are in contact with vascular substance, and where they therefore obtain the freshest cytoblastema."[43] This cytoblastema, which may be minimal in amount, exudes from the vessels into the avascular tissue. In cartilage newly-formed cells sometimes appeared deep within the cartilage substance, far removed from blood vessels. It seemed therefore, "as if cartilage had a greater capacity of imbibition, so that the cytoblastema penetrating from the blood vessels into the parenchyma arrived at the deeper seated portions of the tissue more speedily; and, therefore, retained its fresh plastic force . . . or as if . . . the cytoblastema retained its productive power for a longer period."[44] Cell production required cytoblastema. Cell formation in unusual quantity, or under unusual conditions, could be explained only by assuming an especial "potency" in the blastema or special circumstances under which it operated. Cytoblastema could "explain" any observation, simply by possessing a special power to bring about the datum in question. As we noted earlier, this has descriptive value, for it calls attention to phenomena and observational sequences, but is not a meaningful explanation.

The concept of new cell formation occurring in a blastema raised still further difficulties. Schwann's main thesis was that cells, even though physiologically or functionally very different, all developed in the same manner. Where, then, did specificity enter in? Once formed, the cells differentiated into their specific characters, but how? How was a cartilage cell different from an epidermal cell or a kidney cell? What mechanisms were involved in these differences? The blood vessels had no part in producing specificity, for the vessels merely brought about a "more minute distribution of the nutrient fluid."[45] There had to be other factors.

Schwann wondered whether there might perhaps be something in the blastema itself which provided a specific determinant quality. While studying cells of the "horny tissue," he noted that the nutriment or blastema came from the nearest underlying vascular supply. He wondered "whether this cytoblastema which exudes from the matrix have a specific character, and on that account horn-cells are formed in it." The alternative to a specific local determinant seemed to be some effect exerted "by the plan of the entire organism."[46] Or, phrased differently, perhaps a cell "when once formed, continues to grow by its own individual powers, but is at the same time directed by the influence of the entire organism in such manner, as the design of the whole requires."[47]

Both these alternatives were rather nebulous. That some determinant arose from the blood was conceivable, but if this were the case, then the circulating blood must in some fashion exude a distinct specific substance for each separate tissue. On the other hand, it was possible that the organism as a whole somehow determined the growth of each individual part. But this, while a fine imaginative concept, was not readily demonstrable. It was a long time before further knowledge could partially illumine a murky subject.

Schwann's theory of cell formation illustrates the way pitfalls beset even the conscientious observer. The microscope does not ordinarily indicate *process*. Instead, the observer notes many discrete static forms, and then infers —or constructs—a schema which he believes represents true continuity. This leads to a very widespread fallacy, which I would call, "the fallacy of transitional cases." Schwann, studying the formation of cells, did what innumerable later investigators have also done. He selected many discrete forms and then arranged them in a linear (or perhaps stepwise) series, each member differing from the preceding one by only a small increment. He then asserted that some hypothetical dynamic process was at work, to *propel,* so to speak, the first step in the series, through the entire gamut of changes, until the last stage was reached. Once a group of individuals is arranged in stepwise serial order, each intermediate step is assumed to be a *transition* between a natural predecessor and a natural successor. A dynamic transformation is assumed to pervade the component elements.

Following Schleiden, Schwann described carefully graded steps between naked granules and fully formed cells. On the (fallacious) principle of transitional cases, he asserted that this series represents an active dynamic process, which he elaborated into laws of cell growth. However, his original observations were incorrect, his alleged series of transformations proved imaginary, with no basis in fact, and his "laws" were quite unfounded. "Transitional instances" are indeed a weak reed on which to lean. Nevertheless Schwann had a profound insight into the nature of living organisms, an insight not diminished by errors of detail. Once the basic truth was pointed out, other workers could correct the details.

IV

Schwann had erected his theory on two basic concepts, first, that there existed a matrix or blastema; and second, that out of this matrix cells developed through granule formation. Such a viewpoint encountered many difficulties (which Schwann himself probably did not fully realize), and was eventually discarded, in favor of the doctrine that all cells arose from preexisting cells. Meanwhile, however, the idea of a blastema appealed to numerous earnest workers, among whom were Carl Rokitansky (1804–78), the outstanding Viennese pathologist, and John Hughes Bennett, the eminent Scottish physician (1812–75).

Rokitansky developed the blastema concept into a complete "system," quite comparable to those of the eighteenth century. He approached biological problems as a pathologist, that is, as one who is interested in disease. As a pathologist he was enormously skilful and experienced, extremely competent in observing and describing gross changes. He was not, however, equally skilled in microscopy. Virchow, with considerable justification, emphasized this fact in 1846, in a review[48] of Rokitansky's great *Handbuch.* By the 1840's Rokitansky was already established in an older tradition wherein he had achieved great and deserved success. While he did publish very creditable microscopic studies, nevertheless his thought modes had already been formed in the tradition of gross pathology. In contrast Virchow, a brilliant youth, began his professional career with microscopic investigations, and consequently had a quite different attitude toward pathology.

Rokitansky, keen observer that he was, brought to the autopsy table his own intellectual spectacles that gave an eighteenth-century tint to everything he saw. But Virchow, only half a generation younger, nevertheless participated much more fully in the broad advances of the nineteenth century that we can call the "medical revolution."[49]

Whereas Schwann's studies on the blastema concerned normal tissues, Rokitansky applied the blastema concept to disease. He was especially interested in the processes that he called "new growths." Today this term indicates a neoplasm, but Rokitansky could not adequately distinguish between tumors (neoplasms) and inflammations. He lumped them together into one heap, and believed that all of them, inflammations and tumors, arose from distinct blastemas. "New growth" he considered to be something new or "heterologous," supervening in a tissue and causing changes therein. The source of any such new growth was a blastema, which, thought Rokitansky, arises from the blood. Blastemas are multiple. They can exist in several states, and undergo transformations and alterations. They may be fluid or solid, amorphous or organized. They may or may not produce cells, may or may not develop fibers or blood vessels. Blastemas may be benign or malignant, and Rokitansky discussed at considerable length the distinction between the two. In any such discrimination the microscope was not considered very helpful, despite the anticipations to which the instrument had given rise.[50]

Blastema is inseparable from the concept of *process*. Change was of the very essence. Rarely, as if to prove the rule, a blastema might appear to be inert, that is, simply to exist in the tissues as something static. But this was more apparent than real, for ordinarily the blastema started with a given appearance, and in the course of time ended up as something quite different. Furthermore, separate blastemas might initially seem very much alike, but their future transformations could be very different.

For example, two children may have red swollen throats, with involvement of the tonsils. Each child may exhibit a fibrinous deposit, or exudate. Yet in one case the disease will go on to (what we call) diphtheria, while the other may suffer only from a simple though severe tonsilitis. In these two cases the fibrinous exudates may appear quite similar, but not for long. With the passage of time the two diseases show distinct patterns which permit clin-

198

ical recognition. These clinical patterns, with their variations, may become so familiar that a skilful clinician has little difficulty in diagnosis. But the great problem remains *how to account for that clinical pattern.* We today can invoke specific causative bacteria. Rokitansky would attribute the differences to some basic difference in the blastema.

According to the blastema concept certain constituents passed from the blood into the tissues. Blastemas may remain in their original fluid state or may solidify, and from them will ordinarily develop the formed elements such as granules, nuclei, cells, or fibers. This, of course, was Schwann's view. The fate of blastema is variable. It may remain dormant, or show regressive changes and be absorbed, or it may undergo progressive development into various tissues or substances.[51]

Rokitansky devoted considerable attention to inflammatory exudates. The exuded fibrin might undergo many different transformations. It might remain a simple coagulum, or might give rise to granules and nuclei. It might exhibit "destructive" tendencies or might heal and "convert" into fibrous tissue. The future course of the exudate, as it developed, he regarded as the *property of fibrin itself,* serving to differentiate one kind from another. Since the exudates showed different appearances and underwent different outcomes, he attributed the reason therefore to the specific blastema which the exudate represented. He distinguished "simple" fibrinous forms, as well as other forms such as the croupous, the fibrino-tuberculous, the purulent and ichorous, with their varieties.[52]

Of great importance was the nature of pus. This he considered to be a complex substance, consisting of a fluid part, the "pus-serum," together with formed elements, such as "molecular granules," nuclei, and cells. There might also be, he casually noted, "animalcules, etc." Pure pus was an "albuminous exudate, out of which . . . the pus-cell becomes developed by virtue of a specific conversion."[53] Pus was not, strictly speaking, a blastema. On serous surfaces and within solid tissues, "a solidifying fibrinous blastema is frequently thrown out." Then careful inspection will show pus cells and granules floating in the albuminous fluid, but the pus cells do not develop out of the fibrin exudate but from the "sero-albuminous moisture" which accompanies it.[54] "Normal" pus is quite bland, but "ichor" which "often closely resembles pus in appearance, is distinguished from the bland nature of true pus, by its corroding influence upon the textures [tissues]."[55]

While some exudates were harmless, others were quite the reverse. Many inflammations were severely destructive of tissues. Especially severe were the "croupous" exudates. Rokitansky emphasized the "early tendency to break down" or liquefy, the frequent "corrosive, texture-softening power."[56] In other words, he was describing infectious processes which damaged the tissues and produced ulcerations. He realized that there were certain features in common between, for example, "sloughing tonsils" and "puerperal putrescence of the womb."[57] Without knowing anything about bacteria he clearly realized that some exudates had much in common with each other, and as a class differed from other types of exudate. Each class of exudate, with its characteristic "activity," he denominated as a separate blastema. Each blastema had its own "cause," which we will discuss later.

Rokitansky's doctrines of tuberculosis admirably illustrate the blastema theory. He knew nothing about specific bacteria, and the concepts of virulence and hypersensitivity were equally unknown. For him the tubercle was an "exudate" of characteristic form and appearance, that is, a specific blastema that "persists at the lowest grade of development . . . in the primitive crude condition."[58] He differentiated two types of tubercle, which he called the gray and the yellow. We know today that the gray form represents a simple granuloma without any (significant) necrosis, while the yellow tubercle exhibits caseation, and indicates a hypersensitive state. To Rokitansky, the gray and the yellow tubercles, which we know indicate a difference in host reactivity, represented two distinct blastemas which were usually concurrent. Each had its own range of reaction or development. The gray tubercle either remained as it was, or, if it involuted, dried up into a minute tough mass, or "cornification." On the other hand, the yellow tubercle could enlarge, become soft, confluent, and even progress to complete liquefaction. The softening (caseation) might take place rapidly or slowly, early in the disease or late, and "is a spontaneous metamorphosis essentially proper to the nature of tubercle."[59] However, the yellow tubercle might also show regression, with calcification.

The tuberculous blastemas might coexist with others. "Inflammation" and "fibrosis" represented separate blastemas which can enter into complicated interrelations with "tubercle." When the tuberculosis heals and gives rise to fibrous scars, this fibrosis does not arise from tubercle but from the "organizable blastema, effused together with the tubercle and incorporated in it."[60]

Rokitansky was trying to indicate specificity. He believed there were two distinct and independent basic tuberculous reactions, and indicated this distinction by assigning to each a separate blastema. And repair was quite a different process, entirely distinct from tubercle. Since reparative fibrosis occurs in a wide variety of diseases, there was, he reasonably assumed, a separate blastema which provided repair-characters whenever and wherever required, whether in tuberculosis or abscess or ulceration. *He was trying to isolate units of pathological activity and define the limits for each unit.* He was, as it were, *atomizing* the various pathological activities.

This is especially significant when we consider how very little was then known about cells. To be sure, in the 1840's cells and nuclei were recognized, but there was no identification of specific functional units. Appreciation and clear identification of a fibroblast, a macrophage, a monocyte, a polymorphonuclear leucocyte, were still a long way ahead. Investigators, while they might indeed talk about cells, could not as yet use these cells for predictive or analytical purposes and could not correlate microscopic appearances and grossly observable processes. Rokitansky, therefore, when he wanted to express needed specificity, did so not through cells or microscopy but through *units of process* which he could correlate with gross observations. Blastema was a term which indicated process and specificity, embodied in a visible and grossly recognizable form.

Different blastemas possessed "indwelling properties of their own,"[61] and Rokitansky tried to indicate some of the determining factors and inner mechanisms. Blastemas, in all their variety, were not independent, but represented a more basic condition of the blood. A given blastema reflected a blood state which he called a *crasis:* the numerous and varied exudates—blastemas—stemmed from "the endogenous impairment of the blood within the vascular system." Localized pathologic changes depended on "pre-existing impairment of the general circulation . . . primitive affections of the entire blood mass."[62] This, of course, is humoral pathology at its most vigorous: blood disturbances underlie pathology.

Rokitansky, in assuming the blood to be the ultimate locus of disease states, tried to correlate known differences in the blood with particular disease categories. But how much could he detect in the blood? How many differential features could he identify, which he might correlate with this or that disease? The essential components which he was able to study were the formed elements or blood globules; the fibrin, which coagulated and separated out when the blood no longer circulated; and the albuminous and serous (that is, the non-coagulable liquid) constituents. The available evidence suggested that disturbances in the fibrin were somehow responsible for many different diseases, especially those called "inflammatory." Bronchitis, pneumonia, peritonitis, meningitis, all show inflammatory exudate. It seemed very logical to connect the circulating fibrin of the blood and the fibrin of the various exudates; and to maintain that differences in the disease entity reflect some primary difference in the blood fibrin.

What differences? Anatomical pathology was not adequate to identify any specific factors. Chemistry—chemical pathology—was promising but still inadequate. Chemical analysis, said Rokitansky, could demonstrate some changes, such as the "quanitative excess of fibrin in the blood,"[63] decrease in the blood globules, or increase in fat. But this quantitative variation was not sufficient to achieve any sound correlation with disease states. Repeatedly he emphasized that some qualitative variation was essential. One fibrin-crasis must differ from another by virtue of some *quality* or qualitative feature. What this might be he did not know. Neither anatomy nor chemistry could as yet supply the answer. He urged the "chemical pathologist" to an "unremitting prosecution of his researches to study the ingredients of the blood and the changes these undergo."[64] He declared, somewhat plaintively, that "Investigations are urgently requisite which have for their principal aim to determine the qualitative impairment of the fibrin."[65] We realize today that when pathogenic bacteria were discovered, a large part of his answer was supplied.

The doctrine of crasis found its most convincing support from the infectious diseases. The theory of fibrin-crases tried to correlate clinical disease-states with a hypothetical state of the fibrin. The most primitive form was a "simple" fibrin crasis, involving merely coagulation within vessels, as thrombi. When, however, inflammatory exudates occurred and fibrin was deposited outside the vessels, there was a more "advanced" stage. In a "croupous" crasis the exudate often seemed to exert a "corroding, solvent effect upon the textures [tissues],"[66] even though the reason was not clear. To us this indicates bacterial infection with greater or lesser degree of tissue damage, ulceration, and destruction. There were several distinct subclasses corresponding to clinical features, yet common to all was the fibrinous exudate. The specificity that we attribute to the bacteria he attributed to some special quality in the blood. His doctrine is more plausible if we can substitute "specific bacterium" for "specific quality."

Tuberculosis had its own crasis which, as already discussed, manifested itself in special blastemas. Rokitansky, however, did not believe that tuberculosis could be cured merely by local changes. Healing took place, not on the local level, but only when there is "extinction of the tuberculous crasis" and no "fresh tuberculous matter" is deposited.[67] In other words, true systemic changes underlay any cure, and local progression or regression of the disease merely reflected something more fundamental that was related to "humors."

Rokitansky tried to associate certain disease groups with observable states of the blood. Apart from excess or diminution of fibrin there might, for example, be a "preponderance of blood globules," as in "plethoric" crases; or preponderance of the watery parts, with diminution in fibrin, albumin, and blood globules, as in anemia; or a septic state with "decomposition" of the blood; or crases characterized by retention of urea, or of bile. In large part, however, he was unable to demonstrate any specific blood change. In such instances he could only fall back on faith, faith that there *was* a specific causative factor which resided in the blood, and that future research, especially in chemistry, would demonstrate this factor.

The doctrine of crases, like so much old medical theory, has been discredited. If we want to understand how it went astray, we should seek the implicit assumptions which had been accepted uncritically, and which distorted the measure of truth that may lurk even within error.

The first assumption is a simple question of fact. When Rokitansky alleged a particular change in the blood, was that change "really" present? For example, does a given sample of blood contain an actual excess of fibrin? This might seem a simple problem which, in theory, should permit a yes-or-no answer. But there lies concealed a second assumption, which complicates the question. This may be called the assumption of homogeneity. That is to say, he was taking for granted that what he called fibrin in one case was the same as what he called fibrin in another case. This, of course, was not necessarily so. The term "fibrin," as he used it, included a considerable number of factors which he could not discriminate. In other words, what he believed was a uniform substance turned out later to be quite heterogeneous. Hence, a statement that a sample of blood did or did not contain excess "fibrin" was not useful, until the term "fibrin" was more clearly defined.

The third assumption concerns significance. Supposing that observations are factually correct, we may then ask, are they truly significant? Rokitansky believed that he observed certain changes in the blood in certain disease states. Assuming these to be facts, were they significantly related to the disease process? For example, was an alleged increase in blood fibrin causally related to a pneumonia or a peritonitis? Facts must not be loaded with interpretations they cannot support, nor significance assumed without demonstration.

A fourth assumption deals with unwarranted generalization. A formulation that might be plausible in one context should not be uncritically extended into other areas. A generalization substantially valid within certain limits must not be uncritically applied to areas with quite different characteristics. We may, for example, allow considerable merit to the crasis theory in regard to certain selected infectious diseases. This does not warrant the extension to other and non-infectious diseases.

These assumptions, adopted uncritically, account for much of Rokitansky's error. Frequently he accepted as fact what simply was not so; and he placed heterogeneous states in a single category. He often assumed significance in trivial findings. And he extended his generalizations from one area to another without any specific evidence that such extension was justified.

Rokitansky believed that humoral factors—blood proteins, for example—would explain disease processes. His insights, which at the time were little more than imagination, have after a century and more received surprising support. Even the "cancer crasis," once so roundly condemned, has become very signicant as the humoral aspects of cancer receive more and more attention. Rokitansky had bet heavily on the blood as, somehow, the ultimate explanation in disease. Virchow, as we shall see, had bet on the cells, and superciliously dismissed the humoral factors. In the short run, knowledge of cells far outstripped chemical knowledge about the blood. Virchow seemed for a time to have backed the clear winner. But Rokitansky's horse, although a slow starter, had tremendous stamina, and after a hundred years began at last to reveal excellent form.

V

Virchow was one of the greatest physicians of the nineteenth century, as well as one of the most famous. For both the historian and the general reader the recent biography of Virchow[68] presents a splendid introduction to the man, his work, and his impact on medicine. In the present chapter only a few selected aspects of his doctrines are discussed, with special reference to methodology and cell theory.

In 1846 Virchow emphasized observation and experiment as the basis of a true pathologic physiology, and condemned speculation and hypothesis. His view was that hypothesis had only a transitory value, to serve as the "mother of experiments," that is, to elicit new facts. Hypotheses cannot rest without adequate proof or, in the modern idiom, without verification. Virchow severely criticized Rokitansky and the whole Viennese school for its dogmatism, neglect of adequate proof, and for so intermingling hypotheses and observation that the reader cannot distinguish between them. When available facts are not sufficient, the hiatus, he said, should be filled in with new facts, not with hypotheses.[69] "The hypotheses and analogies in themselves have no value in scientific investigation except . . . that they function as entering wedges for further investigation."[70] He liked to decry speculative thinking and to emphasize the sacredness of facts. In rather windy rhetoric he declared for "the authority of fact, the justification of the particular, and the rule of law."[71]

Despite his unpleasant manners and the wordiness that sometimes bordered on fustian, Virchow was in large part correct. A theory must be well grounded on fact. If facts are insufficient, then speculation and hypothesis can carry on for a while, but unless new and relevant facts are shortly forthcoming, the theory will collapse.

This did indeed happen to the crasis and blastema theory. The chemical study of blood and exudate did not progress very rapidly. Without new data, new concrete evidence, the doctrine was bound to wither. Chemistry did make very substantial progress but not of a sort needed to fill up the holes in the crasis theory. On the other hand the study of cells advanced tremendously. Battalions of eager and able workers provided a wealth of new data. Improved instruments made the task easier. Of course there were abundant errors, but this was only to be expected in a relatively new field.

Schwann's original formulation was rendered untenable. Baker[72] has traced especially well the various points of view in mid-nineteenth-century cell theory. The doctrine which finally prevailed was that all cells arose from other cells, the famous principle *"omnis cellula e cellula,"* that was established principally by Remak (1815–65) and by Virchow. Virchow was by far the more flamboyant, but critical opinion gives essential credit to Remak. Baker compares the two: "Remak was a typical research-worker. He carried out thorough investigations in the laboratory; he studied carefully the work of others, and made full acknowledgment of it; he wrote in a straightforward style and eschewed all fanciful ideas. Virchow, on the contrary, soared away in the manner of his predecessors in the school of *Naturphilosophie,* and left the reader guessing what the actual facts were that led him to his conclusions, and who discovered them."[73] It is an interesting commentary that Virchow, who so prided himself on his scientific method, and criticized everyone else so freely, should be recognized as an offshoot of the very school he condemned. In this connection Pagel's excellent studies[74] on the relation of Virchow to his speculative predecessors should be consulted.

Virchow indeed contributed a great deal that was new in pathology, but perhaps his strength lay in the hard-driving way in which he popularized his beliefs. His great book *Cellular Pathology*[75] disseminated the new doctrines and offers a fine survey of his views. Yet Ackerknecht's comment is relevant, that "The historian is likely to be impressed less by Virchow's discoveries than by his ability to make men accept his ideas."[76] This was a great virtue when his opinions were correct, but when he was in error it was a positive disservice that he rendered. Inasmuch as Virchow acquired a canonical status in pathology, his authority was widely accepted, and his errors were consequently more disastrous.

In the early days of cell theory, the cells could be observed to multiply, but their provenance was at first not clear. That they might develop out of the gelatinous or semifluid matrix in which they were observed, seemed not at all unreasonable. Such development was in essence a "spontaneous" generation: a granule appeared where previously there was none. This granule, it was thought, developed into a nucleus, and then a cell. As we have noted, such a viewpoint did not explain how specificity arose. In pathologic formations Rokitansky attributed the specificity first of all to qualitative differences in the blastema. But since this was itself a derivative, he carried the process a stage further back, and attributed specificity to some particular state of the blood. This was called a crasis, but he did not try to probe its cause.

Virchow started from the opposite direction. Strongly opposed to spontaneous generation, he nevertheless at first adhered to some sort of blastema concept, stating explicitly, in 1847, that all organization takes place by differentiation of a formless blastema.[77] However, as he developed his cellular pathology, he disregarded the blastema and his textbook, in 1858, disclosed his maturer views. Instead of having the cellular elements arise from an intercellular matrix, he reversed the process and made the latter dependent on the cell.

Virchow's protestations about evidence and fact and proof, and his (verbal) abhorrence of speculation are not very convincing. He was a "systematist" just as much as was Rokitansky. That is, they both tried to find an all-inclusive formulation, a formulation based on concrete evidence but elaborated to form a broad imaginative construct. Nevertheless, Virchow as a system-maker had the supreme virtue of being quite close to the truth. He was right, but not because of his scientific method. It is not true that he carefully amassed evidence, exerted impeccable reasoning, used only well-controlled experiments, and built up inductive conclusions in interlocking fashion. This is what Harvey did to prove his contentions. But Virchow was not another Harvey. Rather was he a true descendent of speculative biology, although more disciplined than his predecessors. His speculative insight "paid off" in certain important respects. Starting with a limited amount of evidence he took a tremendous inductive leap —and landed safely. Safely, that is, so far as his main contention is concerned, that cells arise from cells. However, when he tried to elaborate this concept, and use it to "explain" the various pathologic phenomena, he sometimes fell into a morass of error.

Virchow divided the body tissues into three groups, the epithelial structures, the connective tissue elements, and a third more heterogeneous group that included muscles, nerves and vessels.[78] For our purposes the connective tissues are of special interest. Virchow considered the cell as the starting point of biology, and any animal as the sum of its cells. But animals (in contrast to plants) show considerable amounts of intercellular substance, that is, material between cells. He developed a concept of "cell territories," of interstitial material directly dependent on a cell. Where this intercellular material occurred, "every cell, in addition to its own contents, has the superintendence of a certain quantity of matter external to it, and this shares in its changes."[79]

We can, perhaps, continue Virchow's metaphor of "territory," and say that every portion of the body which is not a cell is under the direct "ownership"—control or influence—of some cell. It follows that if there is no "unowned land" independent of cells, then there is no matrix *prior* to cells, out of which a cell can arise. What might seem to be a matrix, the intercellular material that makes up a considerable proportion of the body, is really only a product and not a source.

The locus from which new cells arose was shifted, therefore, from an undifferentiated matrix to pre-existing cells. In normal tissues such as the epidermis or liver it was not difficult to believe that a new cell arose from division of a cell already there. The new cell resembled the old cell. The precise mode of division might not be entirely clear, for the complexities of mitosis had not yet been untangled, but this would be only a detail. However, pathological states produced considerable difficulty, for disease might bring forth new forms quite different from normal elements. Today we can directly observe various cell transformations, but Virchow could not. Technique was not developed to that point. The cells of pus and other new formations had to come from somewhere, and his theory demanded that they come from other cells. He concluded that in large part these new formations arose locally from cells of the connective tissue. Whereas for Rokitansky a formless blastema was the source for new growths, for

Virchow blastema or an exudate were unacceptable. For a blastema he substituted the connective tissue cells.

With but slight limitations we can dismiss the earlier blastema, the later exudate, the primitive plastic lymph of the older authors, and substitute in their place the connective tissue and its equivalents, to serve as the common germinal source for the body, and from this we can derive the actual subsequent developments.[80]

A brief glance at pus and suppuration will help illustrate the development of cell theory. Rokitansky's view we have briefly noted. Virchow set himself against the Viennese pathologist's doctrine, and brought forward data and inferences that are quite interesting. Virchow had devoted considerable study to the blood, and probably his best work was on thrombosis and embolism. He was familiar with the white cells of the blood and was the first to appreciate the real nature of leukemia. The "colorless corpuscles" of the blood he realized were of two types, those with a single nucleus and those with "several" nuclei. The former we know to be lymphocytes, the latter the polymorphonuclear leukocytes, but Virchow could not make this distinction. He believed that a given cell might have one nucleus at an early stage, multiple nuclei later.[81] He appreciated many phenomena of leukocytosis—the rapid increase in circulating leukocytes—and knew that in sedimented blood a layer of white cells formed at the lower part of the buffy coat. The multinucleated colorless corpuscles in the circulating blood he recognized as similar to the corpuscles found in pus. In fact, "a pus-corpuscle can be distinguished from a colourless blood-cell *by nothing else than its mode of origin.*"[82]

According to Virchow, a white cell in the blood stayed in the blood while a white cell found in the tissues *arose locally from the pre-existing tissue cells.* This, in a sense, is the crux of his doctrine. Although other workers had suggested the obvious inference, that the pus corpuscles, so-called, were extravasated blood cells, that is, passed from the circulating blood into the tissues, Virchow expressly rejected this idea.[83] Inflammation, he believed, was a local process, and inflammatory cells and fibrin arose locally.

Virchow, like Rokitansky, was impressed by the varieties of inflammation. The differences Virchow considered to lie not in the blood but in local factors. He thought fibrin formed locally, was absorbed into the lymph and thence into the blood. If the lymph could not remove all the formed fibrin, the surplus constituted the exudate. Increase in fibrin, he noted, was accompanied by increase in white blood corpuscles.

As for the pus-cells—the white corpuscles found in the tissues—he considered that there might be a dual origin, from epithelium or from connective tissue cells. Virchow had to explain the obvious data that some inflammations were associated with ulcerations and necrosis; while others, such as "catarrh," exhibited abundant pus cells but no surface ulcerations. His explanation rested on the basic assumption that cells could readily transform from one type to another. Virchow succumbed to the fallacy of transitional instances. He believed, for example, that a pus cell, a mucus cell and an epithelial cell could be arranged in transitional forms, and that they exhibited intermediate stages. He did not mean that there was a free interchange between these, but that there were primitive undifferentiated cells from which they developed. In epithelium the "very youngest elements . . . cannot be called epithelial cells, or at least they have as yet nothing typical about them, but are indifferent formative cells, which might also become mucus- or pus-corpuscles. Pus-, mucus- and epithelial cells are therefore pathologically equivalent parts which may indeed replace one another, but cannot perform each other's functions."[84]

This quotation deserves a word of comment. First, it was pure hypothesis. Virchow could point to certain cells and he could assert loudly that these gave rise to certain other cells, but this can scarcely be called proof. His assertion does not have much more logical cogency than did Schwann's assertions regarding cell development. Both were hypotheses based on fragmentary evidence. And second, there is great similarity between his concept and a blastema. In each case there was an inferential mother-substance from which various cell-forms differentiated. This mother-substance Rokitansky *called* a blastema; Virchow *called* it an indifferent formative cell. Both were hypotheses. But since Virchow's errors were related to the successful concept *"omnis cellula e cellula,"* they were not as serious as Rokitansky's. Virchow's hypothesis could better accommodate itself to new data and harmonize with later microscopic discoveries.

"As long as the pus is formed out of epithelium, it is naturally produced without any considerable loss of substance and without ulceration."[85] This is his explanation of "catarrh," where there is an exudate but no ulceration. In ulcerative processes the inflammation is more severe and, he thought, pus cells arise from the connective tissue. This may occur with great rapidity. "A single connective-tissue cell may in an extremely short space of time produce some dozens of pus-cells, for the development of pus follows an extremely hurried course."[86] As pus accumulates in the deeper portions, the surface gives way. The epithelium becomes detached, the cells "pour themselves out upon the surface, and a destruction takes place. . . . This is an *ulcer* properly so called."[87]

This is part of his general concept of cell-transformation, which is of even wider extent than inflammation, and applies to many tissues, normal and pathological. For example, he studied bone quite extensively and thought that both cartilage cells and marrow cells could become bone cells.[88] Bone tissue is formed from periosteum, and cartilage and marrow from osseous tissue.[89] And from marrow to fluid is only a "short step," so that there is no sharp boundary between marrow and pus.[90] Pus is not some special product, but can be "traced back to the elements of the pre-existing tissue" in a perfectly regular manner.[91]

The development of cancer he considered to be not dissimilar to that of pus. There was a basic concept of a "heteroplastic process," that is, the process whereby, in any cell proliferation, the new cells showed a change in character from the parent cell. All the various heteroplastic processes, including cancer and tubercle, he considered to be essentially similar, although the various derivatives might show considerable difference in "malignancy."

Virchow believed that cancer arose from the connective tissues. In Figure 138 of his *Cellular Pathology* he illustrated the "transformation" from a "connective tissue corpuscle" to masses of carcinoma cells.[92] His error, of course, derived from inadequate knowledge, hasty generalization on insufficient evidence, and an overweening desire to unify the explanations for various pathologic phenomena. It is of interest that he never finished his great book on tumors,[93] abandoning the work without presenting detailed views on carcinoma. He had already firmly committed himself to certain views that even then were questionable. We can only speculate regarding his failure to publish. Did he suspect that, if he did further work, he would be forced to admit he had been wrong?

Virchow was so concerned with polemics, so driven by the need to argue someone down, that pathology as a science suffered. Even though he undoubtedly was a keen observer, he is scarcely a model for good scientific method.

Perhaps he considered himself much more of a revolutionary than he actually was, and felt some inner urge to magnify the difference between himself and his predecessors (or contemporaries).

In this connection it is interesting to see the persistence of some old ideas. We have already discussed Boerhaave's vascular theories and noted that hypothetical vessels, with hypothetical qualities, were thought to perform functions later attributed to cells. In the nineteenth century the transport function which belonged to a vessel became joined to a particular morphology which belongs to a cell. Virchow, despite his scorn for speculative hypothesis, cultivated this notion. He was always ready to label his opponents' views as vain hypotheses, but found it difficult to see that his own assertions sometimes lacked support.

The problem was another ghost of the blastema theory. We have already seen how Schwann tried to account for the nutrition of non-vascular areas. Cartilage has no vessels, yet it grows and is nourished. Schwann explained this through the hypothesis of an exuded blastema. Virchow rejected the blastema, but he could not so easily explain how tissues with scanty blood supply receive their nourishment. Boerhaave had offered a very straightforward answer: the blood vessels that we can see are continued into myriads of invisible vessels of diminishing caliber. For any tissue there is always an adequate number of vessels but they are invisible. This assertion no one can disprove. It can neither be demonstrated as false, nor shown to be true. The hypothesis, of no cogency, had originally derived from a misinterpretation of observed facts.

Virchow also misinterpreted his observations. When he tried to explain the nourishment of bone, he noted, microscopically, the system of canaliculi, and apparently believed that they were identical with bone cells or bone corpuscles.[94] He thought that these "bone corpuscles" (canaliculi) were connected with one another and with the blood vessels, so that vascular juices which could not permeate the calcareous material, would be "confined to these delicate, continuous, and specially provided channels, and forced to move onwards in canals which are inaccessible to injections from the vessels."[95]

Then, starting with the assumed identity of these canals and the bone cells, he started to generalize. He examined other poorly-vascularized tissues. In fibrocartilage, where vessels are "almost entirely wanting," he noted that the tissues "are pervaded by a fine, stellate system of tubes, or, if you will, of cells, inasmuch as the notion of a tube and that of a cell here quite coincide."[96] He believed that nutrition of cartilage depended on an "ultimate, minute system of cells . . ." and that these ultimate elements "consist of very delicate cells, which are prolonged into fine filaments, that in turn ramify. . . . The filaments can ultimately be very distinctly traced back to the common cell. . . . They are extremely fine tubes . . . connected with one another . . . [and] in certain spots collected into large groups, by means of which the conveyance of the nutritive juice is principally effected. . . ."[97]

He continued his analysis with tendon where, he thought, special stellate cells anastomose with each other, and establish a communication between the vascular and the non-vascular portions, to form a system of juice-carrying canals. By a process of reasoning he concluded that nutritive juices could be distributed only by special canals, and that special cells were the channels for transmission.[98] He also believed that the looser connective tissue had similar systems of tubes, and that elastic fibers were involved. He was not quite sure whether in the transformation of connective tissue cells into elastic fibers the change went so far "as entirely to obliterate their cavity, and thus completely destroy their powers of conduction, or whether a small cavity remains in their interior." He believed that "a very small portion of the cell-cavity remained."[99] In other words, there was a system of fine canals which transported nutritive juices where the ordinary blood capillaries [the "sanguiferous vessels" of Boerhaave] did not extend. These special canals were finer than the capillaries and their locus was in cells.

This, of course, was rather similar, *mutatis mutandis,* to what Boerhaave had claimed. But the "serous vessels" of the older writers Virchow considered to be something merely imagined, "hypothesis" in its most pejorative sense, while he himself was able to offer "something definite."[100] Looking into a microscope, he could point to structures there seen. There is something substantial and reassuringly factual in seeing and pointing to an object. And then it is very easy to endow those objects with properties which are not demonstrated. Virchow baldly asserted that cells observed under the microscope were tubes which conducted nutritive juices. When he said this, he believed that he was demonstrating facts. That he was actually engaging only in speculation and hypothesis did not occur to him. He was often rather insensitive to the distinction between datum and inference.

Early cell theory as propounded by Virchow was essentially a "system," a vast improvement over the eighteenth-century examples but still comparable to them. The amount of available information was relatively small, the number of problems very large. It was not possible to furnish satisfactory, logical, well-grounded explanations for the innumerable puzzling phenomena. But what could not be soundly explained might nevertheless, within the limits of the theory, be subject to conjecture and hypothesis. It is only natural to stretch what information we possess and hope that it will cover the gaps in our present knowledge. While the concept of the cell was a tremendous scientific advance, early cell theory could not meet all the strains that the pulling and stretching entailed. The later development of cell theory into its present form and the integration of many separate disciplines is a fascinating story, but lies outside the scope of this chapter.

With Virchow we enter, for the first time, the modern era of pathology. Despite errors and doubtful logic, his great book, published in 1858, has a modern ring. Many terms that he originated or popularized still find their place in present-day textbooks, and many of his teachings are still entirely acceptable. His basic doctrine represented an insight that proved very fruitful. He was a leader in that company of nineteenth-century giants who laid the foundation for twentieth-century medical achievements.

Epilogue

From the present complexity of medical science it is tempting to look back a hundred years or so as if to a golden age, when knowledge was relatively simple and new discoveries were waiting like ripe peaches to be picked. In retrospect the 1840's and 1850's now seem to be such a period, exciting and full of opportunity. For example, the discovery of cells gave promise of solving nature's mysteries, but it was a promise which was scarcely fulfilled. Study of cell properties raised far more problems than it settled.

Even before the identification of cells, clinicians had been able to describe diseases with considerable accuracy; but when they tried to explain these disorders there was difficulty and confusion. In the earlier chapters we have traced some of these explanatory efforts. Humors and faculties, vital principles and metaphysical concepts, hypothetical structures and mechanical forces, have all had their adherents, and served to bring some sort of order into the baffling flux of phenomena. But the degree of order that any of these could achieve proved inadequate. New explanations succeeded one another, each related to the prevailing conceptual environment, and each seeking greater generality and adequacy relative to medical data.

When at last cells were discovered, a new vista opened up. No longer was it necessary to hypothesize various anatomical structures such as ultimate fibers, particles, and vessels. These had been products of inference, rather than observation, which had given rise to endless controversy but no longer exerted any explanatory force. Instead, investigators had something truly demonstrable to fall back on, something directly visible whose properties could be studied. Metaphysics was to be banished and the age of positivism dawned bright.

The nineteenth century was indeed an era of stupendous progress in medicine. Brilliant clinical observations accompanied great advances in the basic sciences. Cell theory was a major step, but only one among many. When William Osler, in January 1901, reviewed the medical progress of the nineteenth century,[1] he laid special emphasis on bacteriological discoveries and the correlative progress in preventive medicine. When he wrote, bacteriological science had flourished for not much more than a quarter of a century, but its achievements were already highly dramatic. In many infectious diseases a causative microorganism had already been isolated and the whole field of infectious diseases seemed open to conquest. Recognition that bacteria could "cause" disease led to practical advances of extreme importance. Antisepsis and asepsis revolutionized surgery. Knowledge of the sources of infection permitted practical measures to control many diseases.

We might perhaps distinguish between practical and theoretical consequences, even though the two are closely related. The great achievements in asepsis, for example, which with the discovery of anesthesia rendered modern surgery possible, were essentially practical. So too might we construe the conquest of infectious disease through control of the sources of infection, the detection and elimination of carriers or of intermediate hosts. These advances were made possible, however, because bacterial science profoundly affected medical theory. Bacteriology gave precision to the notion of *cause*.

Great physicians, of course, had always concerned themselves with this problem, for it had been obvious that in treating a disease the physician should try to remove the cause. *Tolle causam* had been a watchword since classical times. But the great problem had always been, what *was* the cause? In any rational practice the treatment depended on the answer which the physician gave to these questions. Blind empirical therapy is not an issue here. The great physicians of the past, like those of the present, treated their patients intelligently and rationally. If treatment in earlier periods seems to us quite inappropriate, this means only that the theory on which the treatment was based was incorrect—in other words, that the alleged causes of the disease against which treatment was directed, were wrong. Bacteriological science, however, gave new meaning and significance to the concept "cause of a disease."

It was not enough to find a definite bacterium in a case of any particular disease. The mere presence of a bacterium proved nothing. It was necessary to show a definite relationship, and to demonstrate that a specific bacterium was in fact the cause of a specific disease. Koch discussed the "proof" of a causal relationship between bacterium and disease, and "Koch's postulates" have become a byword in scientific method as applied to medicine.[2] With Koch's postulates the "cause" of a disease began to take on a new significance as something concrete and demonstrable, something without which the disease could not occur. Consequently, once this "cause" was isolated, investigators could, through study of its properties, devise appropriate countermeasures which might cure the patient. Or, in the field of preventive medicine, might avoid infection in the first place.

Of course, as bacteriological discoveries progressed, they raised many new, more complicated, and quite unsuspected problems. Demonstrating the constant presence of a specific bacterium in a specific disease was a fine thing, but why was it that of all people exposed to a specific bacterium, only some individuals contracted the disease? What happened to the bacteria once they entered the body? Why did one patient recover, and another succumb? These and innumerable other questions called for answers. The science of bacteriology expanded to encompass the field called immunology.

The end of the nineteenth century saw the discovery of a new type of infectious agent, the so-called filtrable viruses. Osler, in 1901, could scarcely have predicted the extreme importance that viruses would assume in medical and biological science. Their discovery helped, of course, to untangle the etiology of many specific diseases. But, of even greater importance, the study of viruses has led to greater understanding of biological phenomena and the relationship of chemistry and disease. This understanding is still in an early stage, despite the enormous amount of factual data. The questions that remain unanswered are vastly more numerous and more difficult than those already answered. But one virtue of a new discovery is that it makes possible a new line of questioning, and so opens up new fields of endeavor.

The discovery of virus activity and the realization that

an agent quite different from bacteria was at work, were merely one stage in the development of modern medical theory. There was a great deal of cross-fertilization between one science and another. The data and techniques of many disciplines, apparently quite distinct, were adapted to new goals to achieve new syntheses. Physics, chemistry, and biology were able to assist each other in an unprecedented fashion. Because of this cross-fertilization of sciences, many discoveries have been able to develop to a degree that would have seemed fantastic a century ago.

If Osler were now to look back on the nineteenth century, with the additional perspective of more than sixty years, and knew the advances achieved during this period, he might stress other phases of science, other discoveries of the nineteenth century that have since had profound influence on medical progress. For example, the concepts of evolution, it is now generally agreed, have revolutionized biology to a degree comparable to the sixteenth- and seventeenth-century scientific revolution in physics. Darwin should be ranked with Copernicus, Galileo, and Newton in the influence exerted on subsequent scientific development. And with Darwin we must place Gregor Mendel, whose pioneer achievements in genetics, published obscurely in 1865, remained quite unknown until they were rediscovered in 1900, eighteen years after his death. The science of genetics, with additions from other disciplines, is furnishing a new dimension in medical theory, comparable to what bacteriology had achieved in Osler's day.

The very end of the nineteenth century saw the beginnings of a stupendous advance whose significance Osler could not of course have appreciated. Roentgen and the X-rays, Becquerel, the Curies and radioactivity, have exerted an incalculable effect on medicine. In part this effect has been directly practical. Thanks to the X-ray, every modern practitioner, no matter how mediocre, now

224

has at his command a diagnostic tool superior to what even the most skilful physician possessed seventy-five years ago. And as for treatment, the modern physician, again with the help of X-rays and radium, can achieve therapeutic triumphs that would have seemed impossible a few generations back. The new discoveries in physics around the turn of the century initiated a progress in medicine far more profound than that which followed the adoption of Newtonian physics. We have already noted briefly how Hoffmann and Boerhaave adapted Newtonian doctrines to medical theory. Twentieth-century investigators, like their seventeenth- and eighteenth-century forebears, have also applied physics to biology, but with greater fruitfulness.

In 1901 Osler could scarcely have anticipated the impact that chemistry would have on medical science. Ever since the sixteenth century chemistry had played a significant part in medical practice, and, since the eighteenth century, in medical education as well. The greatest developments were first in the inorganic field where, by the mid-nineteenth century, technique and theory had both expanded markedly. Study of the carbon compounds lagged somewhat, although Wöhler's synthesis of urea in 1828 was an important landmark. What we today call physiological and biochemistry thus had a relatively slower growth than the inorganic aspects. But by the latter part of the nineteenth century progress had been great and the application of chemical science to vital phenomena was becoming extremely important.

Osler appreciated that the training of a good physician should include a sound knowledge of chemistry, physiology, and pathology.[3] By 1900 the textbooks in these subjects contained much chemical information, yet the actual practice of medicine reflected very little thereof. So-called clinical chemistry, the application of chemical analysis to everyday diagnosis and treatment, was extremely rudimentary. The explosive multiplication of knowledge that so completely transformed both theory and practice of medicine did not occur until the twentieth century. Paracelsus, who had dimly realized the significance of chemistry, invoked an "Archeus," which served as an envelope for unknown chemical reactions. Modern investigations into proteins, enzymes, metabolic pathways, oxidation phenomena, energy transformation, and the like, have given a fabulous meaning to the term "Archeus."

Nineteenth-century medical science had become firmly anchored to the cell as the basis for explanation. In the earlier days Schleiden and Schwann were quite unable to offer any satisfactory explanation of how the cells functioned. The proposed "blastema" was a vague and scarcely satisfactory concept, which succumbed to the numerous attacks made upon it. By the 1860's and 1870's sufficient knowledge had accumulated to give a more stable answer. Using microscopes and the knowledge of chemistry then available, the latter nineteenth-century investigators could disregard the blastema and place pathology (the "science of disease") on a firm cellular foundation. But chemistry and physics were achieving fantastic success as both "pure" and "applied" science, and forging techniques that could be applied to other disciplines. The new tools had become so efficient, new concepts so well grounded, that when physics and chemistry, biology and medicine, all interacted, a new level of biological explanation seemed within grasp.

A present-day textbook trying to explain disease goes far beyond the cellular basis as the nineteenth-century physicians understood it. Chemistry, physics and biology have co-operated to offer a deeper insight. Today, more and more, the explanatory terms concern the nature and behavior of such entities as molecules, enzymes, genes, and viruses. The breakdown of complex substances into simpler units, and the converse process of synthesis, have always appealed to theorists. Anaxagoras, as we have already seen, proposed such a scheme in the fifth century B.C. What seemed to be food was actually, he thought, an infinite number of "seeds" which digestive processes separated out, so that they could recombine. And Democritus proposed an atomic theory that was one of the great triumphs in the history of ideas. Modern science is not new in its explanatory scheme of component parts which combine and recombine. What is new is the precise detail and the massive evidence which render inescapable so many of its conclusions.

In biological science, although physics and chemistry have in large part taken over, the cell still remains the focal point. In health and disease the precise details of cellular function, and the correlations between structure and function, are being studied with a fierce intensity. Although much of the latest work is still tentative, the new approach has already borne considerable fruit.

How several disciplines converge to explain a medical problem is brilliantly exemplified in sickle cell anemia, a disease virtually limited to the Negro race. Sometimes red blood cells that appear normal under ordinary circumstance may, when subject to low oxygen tension, assume a peculiar and characteristic "sickle" shape, giving rise to the name "sickle cell." This peculiarity is readily demonstrable by simple techniques. Many Negroes who show no disease symptoms—who in ordinary language are not "sick"—exhibit a certain percentage of red cells of this type. When this property affects some but not all the red cells, it is called the "sickle cell trait," and may cause no overt disturbance. But when virtually all red cells are of this peculiar type, the affected persons exhibit a severe anemia, usually appearing early in life and called "sickle cell anemia." It had long been believed that the disease had a hereditary basis.

Obviously, red cells which became sickled under low oxygen tension were different from those which maintained their normal shape under the same conditions. But what *was* the essential difference? It was Linus Pauling and his co-workers[4] who, in one of the most significant papers of the century, provided the answers. Pauling used the technique of electrophoresis, involving the migration of charged particles in an electric field. The hemoglobin derived from the sickle cells had a different electrophoretic mobility when compared with normals, that is, a different migration rate. Although hemoglobin is a very complex substance, Pauling was able to measure a very exact distinction between the "diseased" form and the normal. The rigidly controlled experiments indicated a precise difference in reaction between the two forms of hemoglobin.

Genetic studies had already suggested that sickle cell anemia represented a homozygous manifestation of a gene which, when heterozygous, yielded the sickle cell trait. Pauling, after identifying the two kinds of hemoglobin, could show that the heterozygote has about 40 per cent of "sickling" hemoglobin, while the homozygote has 100 per cent. The normal person has none. Pauling concluded, "This investigation reveals, therefore, a clear case of change produced in a protein molecule by an allelic change in a single gene involved in synthesis."[5] In the title of his paper Pauling aptly used the term "molecular disease." He had indeed firmly established the disease on a molecular basis.

That a specific gene was responsible for a specific chemical reaction was a relatively new concept, stemming from the work of Beadle and his co-workers.[6] While hereditary diseases had long been recognized, and in many the genetic relationships well worked out, the exact correlation of a particular gene with a particular chemical reaction was first demonstrated by Beadle and associates. They examined the fungus *Neurospora* which possesses a relatively simple genetic structure. By studying mutant strains they showed that the utilization of specific nutritive substances correlated with specific genes. The mutant strains differed from the type by a single gene only. In the absence of a particular gene, a particular chemical reaction concerned with nutrition could not occur. This indicated a strict correlation between gene and enzymatic reaction. Said Beadle, "The inactivation of specific genes is equivalent to the chemical poisoning of specific enzymes." But the genic defect is completely specific while methods which "poison" the enzymes "are often discouragingly non-specific."[7]

In sickle cell anemia a specific gene controls the formation of "sickle" hemoglobin in place of the normal. The next step was to indicate the exact chemical difference between the two hemoglobins and thus pinpoint the activity of the gene in question. Using an ingenious technique, Ingram[8] broke down the hemoglobin molecule and separated the globin moiety into polypeptide chains. The normal and the sickle hemoglobins were the same except for one peptide, which contained eight amino acids. Seven of the eight were identical in the two hemoglobins, but the eighth was different. In the normal hemoglobin it was glutamic acid, in the sickle form it was valine. Thus, among 280 amino acids linked together in a definite pattern, there was a single substitution in a specific locus, which distinguished the sickle hemoglobin from the normal. And in the construction of the hemoglobin molecule a single gene determined this specific substitution. This single difference, a single amino acid substitution, determined by a single gene, was the factor responsible for the entire disease as clinically manifest.

The basic distinction in the sickle hemoglobin gives rise to many derivative characteristics, such as changes in solubility and viscosity in the reduced state. There is increased breakdown of the red cells, leading to the many clinical features which as secondary effects constitute the clinical entity—sickle cell anemia.

As might be expected, the basic discoveries stimulated an enormous amount of work which in turn revealed surprising complexities. There were discovered many different kinds of hemoglobin under genic control. New and unsuspected combinations were identified. These led to re-examination of clinical entities, in the light of the new etiological concepts. The abnormal hemoglobins became a whole scientific realm in their own right. [9]

These abnormal hemoglobins formed merely one area of disease for which a molecular pathology could be established. Defects in other blood constituents were brought into the same rubric, as well as many diseases of varied types. In all of these, some defective molecular behavior can be specifically identified. A molecule may be put together in an "atypical" fashion; some components normally present may be totally absent; or whole molecules may be missing. Many metabolic pathways may exhibit such disturbances. A precise chemical defect may be demonstrable through some highly specific functional disturbance where, for example, a metabolic reaction which takes place normally fails to take place in the diseased individual. A "normal" biochemical reaction may be impeded at one specific locus. Clearly, a specific reaction under enzyme control cannot occur if that enzyme is absent. In a complicated series of metabolic changes the absence of one highly specific enzyme reaction thus *constitutes* the disease. This absence seems to be under genic control. A large number and variety of such conditions exist, for details of which the reader is referred to recent comprehensive expositions.[10]

Explaining disease on a molecular level is still in its early phases, but such an explanation marks a tremendous advance over the cellular pathology of fifty years ago. Cells no longer have quite the significance as *units* that they once held. As cell function was studied more and more minutely, investigators couched their explanations in smaller and more subtle units. Modern physical and chemical techniques have begun to deal effectively with molecular reactions within the cell, in both the cytoplasm and the nucleus.[11] At the same time new anatomical studies are rapidly expanding our knowledge. New techniques are disclosing the ultra-microscopic structure of cells, furnishing concrete morphological data which in time may integrate closely with the newer chemical knowledge. With the electron microscope, cell constituents like mitochondria, long recognized but poorly understood, are assuming new significance. And new techniques of cell dissection allow direct chemical studies on specific cell components.

The present era of medical research is exciting and challenging, yet the pattern of investigation remains essentially the same as in centuries past. Trained workers make observations, draw inferences, and derive concepts which will explain the observations. Throughout history new techniques have made possible new and progressively more subtle observations, greater discrimination and more precise analysis. Thus new data are furnished which are a touchstone for older concepts, and also the raw material for newer and more comprehensive theories. The fresh point of view which new theories engender will give rise to new methods, which in turn lead to progressively greater discrimination in a never-ending cycle. However, the course is never quite orderly. Progress does not follow the naïve Baconian type of induction. Instead, an imagina-

231

tive construct will usually precede the data which validate it. A "hunch" may direct the researcher toward new factual discrimination, or may suggest new ways to discover facts which the hunch had implied.

Observation and theory intermingle and continuously interact, yet constantly progress toward greater complexity. What seemed simple proves to be intricate, what seemed unitary turns out to be composite. A disease category, once "explained" by simple concepts, becomes differentiated into multiple conditions, based on finer discriminations and newly-implicated factors. This is readily apparent if we compare medical textbooks of 1900 and 1962. In any disease category the enormous amount of new observations accumulated over the years could be rendered orderly only by conceptual innovations—new causes, new definitions, new theories, and new disease entities.

All theories have a life history. They start tentatively, grow piecemeal, and slowly become mature. Then they can successfully handle new facts and also have considerable predictive value. But sooner or later a discrepancy appears between facts and theory. Then the theory will become modified, perhaps will entirely disintegrate, to be succeeded by something new.

In this book we have noted a few of the medical theories that were significant in times past. For 2,500 years physicians have tried to explain disease, first by analyzing the elements which composed the body, and then by indicating how diseases result when the elements are somehow disturbed. While this is the over-all pattern of successive medical explanations, the alleged elements have varied widely. The humors of the body, the emanations of the stars, the hard particles bouncing in a mechanical dance, the "least fiber" and the "least vessel," all have had their adherents, as have the "faculties" and the "archei." All these were concepts based on evidence, but perhaps not on very firm evidence. Nevertheless, the physician hypothesized how changes in these entities might account for any particular disease.

However, as science progressed, the canons of evidence became more rigorous and the explanations had to be more exact. We already have noted the great advances which cell theory introduced. But this level of explanation, well grounded as it is, no longer offers sufficient precision. Still smaller units are necessary. These, however, must be very firmly substantiated, since to merit serious attention modern theories must face extremely critical standards.

Present-day medicine has successfully described and explained many diseases in molecular terms. Yet what may fairly be called the molecular theory of disease is still very young, with much progress still to be made. We can be certain that, considering the current rapidity of investigation, this approach to medicine will achieve tremendous success. But the lesson we learn from history is that eventually, after achieving full maturity, this theory will crumble away, and prove quite inadequate. To explain the data eventually to be discovered, new concepts, at present unsuspected, will be suggested. At different periods of history the physician was quite sure that at last he had firmly grasped the truth. Yet invariably he changed his mind. We can be perfectly sure that, despite the marvelous progress of the twentieth century, he will continue to change his mind.

Notes

PROLOGUE

1. Basil Willey, *The Seventeenth Century Background* (London: Chatto & Windus, 1957), pp. 2–3.

CHAPTER I. FROM RELIGION TO SCIENCE

1. Homer, "The Iliad," translated by Andrew Lang, Walter Leaf, and Ernest Myers, *The Complete Works of Homer* (New York: Modern Library).
2. Charles-Victor Daremberg, *La Médicine dans Homère* (Paris: Didier et Cie., 1865), p. 92.
3. Ernest Nagel, *The Structure of Science: Problems in the Logic of Scientific Explanation* (London: Routledge & Kegan Paul, 1961).
4. Emma J. Edelstein and Ludwig Edelstein, *Asclepius: A Collection and Interpretation of the Testimonies* (2 vols.; Baltimore: Johns Hopkins Press, 1945).
5. *Ibid.*, II, 53.
6. *Ibid.*, I, 231–36.
7. *Ibid.*, p. 251.
8. *Ibid.*, pp. 252–53.

9. Ludwig Edelstein, "Greek Medicine in Its Relation to Religion and Magic," *Bulletin of the Institute of the History of Medicine*, V (1937), 201.
10. W. H. S. Jones (trans.), *Hippocrates* (4 vols.; London: Heinemann, 1923–31), I, xxviii.
11. John Chadwick and W. N. Mann (trans.), "Epidemics I," *The Medical Works of Hippocrates* (Oxford: Blackwell, 1950), p. 51. All translations of Hippocrates, unless otherwise indicated, are from this edition.
12. "Epidemics III," pp. 79–80.
13. "Prognosis," pp. 112–13.
14. *Ibid.*, p. 114.
15. *Henry V*, Act II, scene 3.
16. "Aphorisms," p. 166.
17. *Ibid.*, p. 168.
18. *Ibid.*, p. 173.
19. "Prognosis," pp. 117, 124–25.
20. "Aphorisms," p. 171.
21. "Science of Medicine," p. 87.
22. *Ibid.*, pp. 88–89.
23. *Ibid.*, p. 89.
24. "Airs, Waters, Places," p. 94.
25. "Aphorisms," p. 167.
26. "Airs, Waters, Places," pp. 104–9.
27. "Tradition in Medicine," p. 23.
28. "The Nature of Man," p. 204.
29. Sir T. Clifford Albutt, *Greek Medicine in Rome* (London: Macmillan & Co., 1921), p. 99.
30. "The Nature of Man," p. 205.
31. *Ibid.*, p. 207.
32. *Ibid.*, p. 204.
33. "The Sacred Disease," Jones, *op. cit.*, II, 157.
34. *Ibid.*, p. 155.
35. In this connection the Hippocratic text "On Breath" (Jones, II, 251) suggests a somewhat different pathogenesis.
36. "The Sacred Disease," Chadwick and Mann, p. 185.
37. *Ibid.*, p. 186.
38. Chadwick and Mann, pp. 19–26.
39. *Ibid.*, pp. 176–83.
40. "Regimen in Acute Diseases," p. 130.
41. "The Science of Medicine," pp. 82–83.
42. "Tradition in Medicine," p. 12.
43. "The Science of Medicine," p. 83; see also p. 12.
44. *Ibid.*, p. 84.
45. "Tradition in Medicine," p. 17.
46. Owsei Temkin, "Greek Medicine as Science and Craft," *Isis*, XLIV (1953), 211.
47. *Metaphysics* i. l. 981a 6 (Loeb edition).

48. *Ibid.*, i. l. 981a 7–12.
49. "Aphorisms," p. 148.
50. *Metaphysics* i. l. 981a 30–981b 7.
51. *Ibid.*, 981a 27–30.
52. *Ibid.*, 993b 20–23.
53. *Ethica Nicomachea* vi. 2. 1139b 20–25.
54. *Metaphysics* vi. l. 1026a 7–23.

CHAPTER II. SOPHISTICATION

1. R. O. Moon, *The Relation of Medicine to Philosophy* (London: Longmans, Green & Co., 1909), p. 15.
2. George Sarton, *Galen of Pergamon* (Lawrence, Kan.: University of Kansas Press, 1954), p. 51. Italics mine.
3. *Ibid.*, p. 60.
4. "De l'utilité des parties du corps humain," *Oeuvres anatomiques, physiologiques et médicales de Galien,* translated by Charles Daremberg (2 vols.; Paris: J. B. Baillière, 1854), I, 295. (Hereafter referred to as "Daremberg.")
5. Sarton, *op. cit.*, p. 53.
6. Leonard G. Wilson, "Erasistratus, Galen, and the *Pneuma,*" *Bulletin of the History of Medicine,* XXXIII (1959), 293.
7. Daremberg, I, 295; *On the Natural Faculties,* translated by Arthur John Brock, (London: Heinemann, 1952), p. 315. (Hereafter referred to as "Brock.")
8. Daremberg, I, 414, 443; Brock, p. 321.
9. Donald Fleming, "Galen on the Motions of the Blood in the Heart and Lungs," *Isis,* XLVI (1955), 14; Wilson, *op. cit.*; A. Rupert Hall, "Studies on the History of the Cardiovascular System," *Bulletin of the History of Medicine,* XXXIV (1960), 391.
10. Daremberg, I, 381.
11. Wilson, *op. cit.*, p. 313.
12. Daremberg, I, 381.
13. *Ibid.*, p. 437.
14. Brock, p. 323; Daremberg, I, 443.
15. Brock, p. 223.
16. Quoted by Wilson, *op. cit.*, p. 304.
17. Brock, p. 317.
18. Daremberg, I, 406.
19. *Ibid.*, p. 445; Brock, pp. 321–23.
20. Wilson, *op. cit.*, p. 310, points out that Galen did not understand the laws governing flow of liquids through tubes, and that higher pressures in the pulmonary artery can move a larger volume.
21. Brock, p. 321.
22. Daremberg I, 414, 443; Brock, pp. 317, 321.
23. Brock, p. 321.
24. In this connection see Owsei Temkin, "A Galenic Model for Quantitative Physiological Reasoning?" *Bulletin of the History of Medicine,* XXXV (1961), 470.

25. John Burnet, *Early Greek Philosophy* (2d ed.; London: A. and C. Black, 1908), p. 77.
26. Aristotle *De generatione et corruptione* ii. 6. 333b 15.
27. Burnet, *op. cit.*, p. 240.
28. Cyril Bailey, *The Greek Atomists and Epicurus* (Oxford: Clarendon Press, 1928).
29. *Physica* i. 4. 187a 26–187b 17.
30. Bailey, *op. cit.*, p. 36.
31. *Ibid.*, p. 37.
32. *Ibid.*, p. 39.
33. *Ibid.*, pp. 39–40.
34. Quoted in Burnet, p. 301.
35. *De generatione et corruptione* ii. 3. 330b 3–22.
36. *Ibid.*, 330b 4–6.
37. *Ibid.*, ii. 2. 330a 25–ii. 3. 331b 1.
38. Brock, pp. 195–97; see also p. 139.
39. *Ibid.*, p. 257.
40. *Ibid.*, p. 253.
41. *Ibid.*, p. 241.
42. Galen, "Des Habitudes," in Daremberg, I, 102; see also "On Habits," in Brock, *Greek Medicine* (London and Toronto: J. M. Dent & Sons, 1929), p. 186.
43. Brock (1952), p. 255.
44. *Ibid.*, p. 251.
45. Daremberg, I, 324–25.
46. Brock (1952), pp. 237–39; Daremberg, I, 311.
47. Daremberg, I, 304–7.
48. Brock (1952), pp. 39–41.
49. *Ibid.*, pp. 229–37.
50. *Ibid.*, p. 245.
51. *Ibid.*, pp. 319, 318 n.
52. *Ibid.*, p. 17.
53. *Ibid.*, p. 75.
54. *Ibid.*, p. 87.
55. *Ibid.*, p. 85.
56. *Ibid.*, p. 89.
57. Regarding this problem see note 24 above.
58. Brock (1952), p. 93.
59. *Ibid.*, pp. 101–5; Daremberg, I, 353–54.
60. Brock (1952), pp. 11–13.
61. *Ibid.*, pp. 51–61.
62. *Ibid.*, p. 279.
63. *Ibid.*, p. 69.
64. *Ibid.*, p. 63.
65. *Ibid.*, p. 183.

CHAPTER III. THE PHILOSOPHIC APPROACH

1. John Baptista van Helmont, *Oriatrike, or Physick Refined,* translated by J. C. (London: Lodowick Loyd, 1662), p. 230.
2. R. James, *A Medicinal Dictionary* (3 vols.; London: T. Osborne, 1743), I, lxxxvii.
3. Owsei Temkin, "The Elusiveness of Paracelsus," *Bulletin of the History of Medicine,* XXVI (1952), 201.
4. Charles Daremberg, *Histoire des sciences médicales* (2 vols.; Paris: J. B. Baillière et Fils, 1870), I, 388, 394, 404, 421, and *passim.*
5. Kurt F. Leidecker (trans.), Paracelsus, "Volumen medicinae paramirum" (Supplements to *Bulletin of the History of Medicine* [Baltimore: Johns Hopkins Press, 1949]), pp. iii–iv.
6. Wallace K. Ferguson, *The Renaissance in Historical Thought* (Cambridge, Mass.: Houghton Mifflin Co., 1948).
7. George Sarton, "Science in the Renaissance," *The Civilization of the Renaissance* (New York: Frederick Ungar Publishing Co., 1959), p. 75; Ralph M. Blake, "Natural Science in the Renaissance," in Ralph M. Blake, Curt J. Ducasse, and Edward H. Madden, *Theories of Scientific Method: The Renaissance through the Nineteenth Century* (Seattle: University of Washington Press, 1960), p. 3.
8. A. C. Crombie, *Augustine to Galileo* (London: Falcon Press, 1952); *Robert Grosseteste and the Origins of Experimental Science, 1100–1700* (Oxford: Clarendon Press, 1953).
9. Lynn Thorndike, *A History of Magic and Experimental Science* (8 vols.; New York: Columbia University Press, 1923–58), V, 620.
10. Aristotle *Metaphysics* xii. 7. 1072*a* 26–27.
11. *Ibid.* 1072*b* 4.
12. Walter Pagel, *Paracelsus, An Introduction to Philosophical Medicine of the Renaissance* (Basel: S. Karger, 1958), p. 84. In connection with the philosophy of Paracelsus, in many different aspects, special reference must be made to Pagel, "Paracelsus and the Neoplatonic and Gnostic Traditions," *Ambix,* VIII (1960), 125; and to "The Prime Matter of Paracelsus," *ibid.,* IX (1961), 117.
13. Plotinus, *The Enneads,* translated by Stephen MacKenna (2d ed.; London: Faber & Faber, n.d.), v. 1. 7 (p. 376).
14. *Ibid.,* iv. 8. 6 (p. 362).
15. *Ibid.,* iv. 3. 4 (p. 263).
16. *Ibid.,* iv. 3. 9 (p. 268).
17. *Ibid.,* iv. 3. 17–18 (pp. 274–75); v. 2. 2 (p. 381); ii. 1. 5 (p. 83).
18. Arthur O. Lovejoy, *The Great Chain of Being* (Cambridge, Mass.: Harvard University Press, 1957).
19. William A. Heidel, *Hippocratic Medicine: Its Spirit and Method* (New York: Columbia University Press, 1941), pp. 22–23; Sir William Dampier, *A History of Science* (New York: Macmillan Co., 1935), p. 88; and W. H. S. Jones, "Philosophy and Medicine in Ancient Greece" (Supplements to *Bulletin of the History of Medicine* [Baltimore: Johns Hopkins Press, 1946]), p. 5.

20. Fairly popular accounts of the Cabala may be found in the *Encyclopaedia Britannica* (13th ed.; London: 1926, article "Kabbalah"), and in Henry Morley, *The Life of Henry Cornelius Agrippa von Nettesheim* (2 vols.; London: Chapman and Hall, 1856). For more profound study, reference may be made to Pagel's *Paracelsus,* (1958) and the articles in *Ambix,* reference No. 12, above.

21. Thorndike, *op. cit.*

22. Henry Cornelius Agrippa of Nettesheim, *Three Books of Occult Philosophy,* translated by J. F. (London: Gregory Moule, 1651), p. 2.

23. *Ibid.,* p. 24.

24. *Ibid.,* p. 29. In this quotation "jeat" translates the Latin *belagius;* "aetites," transliterating the Latin, is a stone supposedly found in an eagle's nest; "thunders" translates *tonitrua excitat;* "helatropium" refers to the striped jasper, heliotropium. Cf. Agrippa, *De occulta philosophia libri tres* (Coloniae, 1533), p. 17.

25. "Longa experientia plus quam ratione indagine," *De occulta,* p. 13.

26. *Ibid.,* pp. 26–27.

27. *Ibid.,* pp. 65–66.

28. D. P. Walker, *Spiritual and Demonic Magic from Ficino to Campanella* (London: Warburg Institute, University of London, 1958), pp. 3–60.

29. Agrippa, *op. cit.* (1651), p. 74.

30. *Ibid.,* pp. 32–33.

31. Ficino, quoted by Walker, *op. cit.,* p. 13.

32. Agrippa, *op. cit.* (1533), p. 19.

33. E. R. Dodds, "The Astral Body in Neoplatonism," Appendix II in *Proclus, The Elements of Theology—A Revised Text With Translations, Introductions, and Commentary.* (Oxford: The Clarendon Press, 1933), pp. 313–21; see also Pjlotinus, *op. cit.,* iv. 3. 15 (p. 273).

34. In this connection, see F. Sherwood Taylor, "The Idea of the Quintessence," in *Science, Medicine and History,* ed. E. Ashworth Underwood (2 vols.; London: Oxford University Press, 1953), I, 247.

35. Arthur Edward Waite (trans.), *The New Pearl of Great Price* (London: James Elliott & Co., 1894), p. 160.

36. Agrippa, *op. cit.* (1651), p. 33.

37. Edmund O. von Lippmann, *Einstellung und Ausbreitung der Alchemie* (Berlin: Julius Springer, 1919).

38. H. Stanley Redgrove, *Alchemy, Ancient and Modern* (2d and rev. ed.; London: William Rider & Son, 1922), p. 1.

39. C. G. Jung, *Psychology and Alchemy,* translated by R. F. C. Hull (London: Routledge & Kegan Paul, 1953), p. 217.

40. *New Pearl of Great Price,* p. 96.

41. *Ibid.,* pp. 92–94. In reference to Petrus Bonus, see Thorndike, *op. cit.,* III, 160–61.

42. Redgrove, *op. cit.,* pp. 10–11.

43. Thorndike, *op. cit.*, IV, chaps. xxxviii, liii; V, chap. xxiv.
44. Crombie, *Augustine to Galileo, passim.*
45. Pagel, *Paracelsus*, pp. 258–72; *Ambix, loc. cit.*
46. Robert P. Multauf, "John of Rupescissa and the Origin of Medical Chemistry," *Isis*, XLV (1954), 359; "Medical Chemistry and 'The Paracelsians,' " *Bulletin of the History of Medicine*, XXVIII (1954), 101; "The Significance of Distillation in Renaissance Medical Chemistry," *ibid.*, XXX (1956), 329.
47. Taylor, *op. cit.*
48. Walker, *op. cit.*, pp. 43, 48.
49. Kurt Quecke, "Die Signaturenlehre im Schriftum des Paracelsus," *Beiträge zur Geschichte der Pharmazie und ihrer Nachbargebiete.* (Beiheft der Pharmazie), II, (1955), pp. 41–52.
50. Pagel, *Paracelsus, op. cit.*
51. Paracelsus, "Labyrinthus Medicorum Errantium," in *Medizinische, naturwissenschaftliche und philosophische Schriften*, ed. Karl Sudhoff (14 vols.; I–V, X–XIV, Munich and Berlin: R. Altenbourg, 1928–33; VI–IX, Munich: O. W. Barth, 1922–25), XI, 171–72.
52. *Ibid.*, "Das Buch Paragranum," VIII, 140.
53. *Ibid.*, p. 147.
54. *Ibid.*, pp. 147–49.
55. "Labyrinthus," pp. 175–76.
56. "Paragranum," pp. 183–84.
57. Lester S. King, "Plato's Concepts of Medicine," *Journal of the History of Medicine*, IX (1954), 38.
58. "Labyrinthus," p. 209.
59. Thorndike, *op. cit.*, IV, 530–41; Walker, *op. cit.*, pp. 54–60.
60. "Paragranum," p. 183.
61. "Volumen Medicinae Paramirum," translated Leidecker, *loc. cit.*, p. 18.
62. "Paragranum," p. 183.
63. "Labyrinthus," p. 188.
64. "Volumen Paramirum," (Leidecker), p. 25.
65. *Ibid.*, p. 27.
66. *Ibid.*, p. 26.
67. *Ibid.*, p. 29.
68. *Ibid.*, p. 31.
69. "Labyrinthus," p. 186.
70. *Ibid.*, p. 190; see also "Paragranum," p. 181.
71. "Labyrinthus," p. 187.
72. "Paragranum," pp. 183–84.
73. *Ibid.*, p. 185.
74. "Neun Bücher Archidoxis," III, 118.
75. *Ibid.*, p. 135.
76. Ernst Darmstaedter, "Arznei und Alchemie: Paracelsus-studien," *Studien zur Geschichte der Medizin*, XX (1931), 34.
77. "Paragranum," p. 162.
78. "Volumen Paramirum," (Leidecker), p. 20.

79. *Ibid.*, p. 21.
80. "On the Miners' Sickness," translated by George Rosen in *Four Treatises By Paracelsus,* ed. Henry E. Sigerist, (Baltimore: Johns Hopkins Press, 1941), p. 59.
81. Pagel, *Paracelsus,* p. 91. See also pp. 112, 227–28; and *Ambix* (1961).
82. "On the Miners' Sickness," p. 58.
83. "Labyrinthus," pp. 201–2; "Paragranum," pp. 177–78.
84. George Rosen, *The History of Miners' Diseases: A Medical and Social Interpretation* (New York: Abelard-Schuman, 1943), p. 71.
85. "Die drei (vier) Bücher des Opus Paramirum," IX, 123.
86. *Ibid.*, pp. 123–26.
87. *Ibid.*, p. 123.
88. *Ibid.*, p. 129.
89. *Ibid.*, p. 132.
90. *Ibid.*, pp. 138–39.
91. *Ibid.*, p. 140.
92. *Ibid.*, pp. 141–42.
93. *Ibid.*, p. 143.
94. "On the Miners' Sickness," p. 57.
95. *Ibid.*, pp. 58–59.
96. *Ibid.*, p. 60.
97. *Ibid.*, p. 62.
98. *Ibid.*, pp. 69–71.
99. *Op. cit.*
100. "Opus Paramirum," IX, 45–47.
101. See Pagel, *Paracelsus,* p. 103.
102. "On the Miners' Sickness," p. 64.
103. *Ibid.*, p. 65.
104. *Ibid.*, p. 66.
105. *Ibid.*, p. 85.

CHAPTER IV. PROGRESS AND PITFALLS

1. A. Wolf, *A History of Science, Technology, and Philosophy in the 16th and 17th Centuries* (2d ed.; London: Allen & Unwin, 1950); *ibid., A History of Science, Technology and Philosophy in the Eighteenth Century* (2d ed.; London: Allen & Unwin, 1952); Herbert Butterfield, *The Origins of Modern Science, 1300–1800* (London: G. Bell & Sons, 1951); F. Sherwood Taylor, *A Short History of Science and Scientific Thought* (New York: W. W. Norton & Co., 1949); Marie Boas, "The Establishment of the Mechanical Philosophy," *Osiris,* X (1952), 412–541; A. C. Crombie, *Augustine to Galileo: The History of Science, A.D. 400–1650* (London: Falcon Educational Books, 1952); L. W. H. Hull, *History and Philosophy of Science* (London: Longmans, 1959); William P. D. Wightman, *The Growth of Scientific Ideas* (New Haven: Yale University Press, 1953); A. R. Hall, *The Scientific Revolution, 1500–1800* (Boston:

The Beacon Press, 1956); E. J. Dijksterhuis, *The Mechanizations of the World Picture,* translated by C. Dikshoorn (Oxford: Clarendon Press, 1961); Alexander Koyré, *From the Closed World to the Infinite Universe* (Baltimore: Johns Hopkins Press, 1957).

2. Antonio Benivieni, *De abditis nonnullis ac mirandis morborum et sanationum causis,* translated by Charles Singer (Springfield, Ill.: Charles C Thomas, 1954).
3. *Ibid.,* Case 9, pp. 37–41.
4. *Ibid.,* Case 26, p. 71.
5. *Ibid.,* Case 28, p. 75; Case 30, p. 77.
6. *Ibid.,* Case 25, p. 69.
7. *Ibid.,* Cases 34, 36, pp. 83, 85.
8. Charles Singer, *A Short History of Anatomy from the Greeks to Harvey* (New York: Dover Publications, 1957), p. 77.
9. Charles Singer and C. Rabin, *A Prelude to Modern Science* (Cambridge: University Press, for the Wellcome Historical Medical Museum, 1946), p. ii.
10. L. R. Lind (trans.), Jacopo Berengario da Carpi, *A Short Introduction to Anatomy (Isagogae Breves)* (Chicago: University of Chicago Press, 1959), p. 33. See also Singer and Rabin, *loc. cit.*
11. B. Farrington, "The Preface of Andreas Vesalius to *De fabrica corporis humani* 1543," *Proceedings of the Royal Society of Medicine,* XXV (1932), p. 1361.
12. Singer and Rabin, *op. cit.,* p. xvi.
13. J. B. de C. M. Saunders and Charles D. O'Malley, *The Illustrations from the Works of Andreas Vesalius of Brussels* (Cleveland and New York: World Publishing Co., 1950), p. 42.
14. *Ibid.,* p. 9.
15. Farrington, *op. cit.,* p. 1360.
16. C. E. Kellett, "Sylvius and the Reform of Anatomy," *Medical History,* V (1961), 105.
17. Singer, *op. cit.;* M. F. Ashley Montagu, "Vesalius and the Galenists," in *Science, Medicine, and History,* ed. E. Ashworth Underwood (2 vols.; London: Oxford University Press, 1953), I, 374; Lind, *op. cit.;* Lynn Thorndike, *A History of Magic and Experimental Science* (8 vols.; New York: Columbia University Press, 1923–58), V, 498; Gernot Rath, "Pre-Vesalian Anatomy in the Light of Modern Research," *Bulletin of the History of Medicine,* XXXV (1961), 142; Kellett, *op. cit.*
18. Max Fisch, "Vesalius and His Book," *Bulletin of the Medical Library Association,* XXXI (1943), 208; Rath, *op. cit.;* Saunders and O'Malley, *op. cit.;* Singer and Rabin, *op. cit.;* M. Roth, *Andreas Vesalius Bruxellensis* (Berlin: Reiner, 1892); the forthcoming biography by O'Malley will be eagerly awaited.
19. Thorndike, *op. cit.,* V, 500.
20. Quoted by Montagu, *op. cit.,* p. 377.
21. "Quicumque igitur vult operum naturae esse contemplator, non opportet eum anatomicis libris credere, sed propriis oculis." Galen,

"De Usu Partium," II, 3, in *Opera Omnia*, ed. C. G. Kühn (20 vols. in 22 parts; Leipzig: Cnobloch, 1821–33), III, 98.

22. Singer and Rabin, *op. cit.;* Lind, *op. cit.;* Kellett, *op. cit.;* Rath, *op. cit.*
23. Quoted in Rath, *op. cit.,* p. 148.
24. Singer and Rabin, *op. cit.,* pp. xxxv, lxiii.
25. Fisch, *op. cit.,* p. 213.
26. Singer and Rabin, *op. cit.*
27. Saunders and O'Malley, *Andreas Vesalius Bruxellensis: The Blood-letting Letter of 1539. An Annotated Translation and Study of the Evolution of Vesalius' Scientific Development* (New York: Henry Schumann, n.d.), p. 18.
28. Fisch, *op. cit.,* p. 214.
29. Montagu, *op. cit.,* p. 383.
30. Francis Bacon, "Novum Organum," Book I, Aphorism 82, in *The Works of Francis Bacon* (3 vols.; Philadelphia: Parry & McMillan, 1859), III, 357; Edwin A. Burtt (ed.), *The English Philosophers from Bacon to Mill* (New York: The Modern Library, 1939), p. 57. The quotation as it appears in the text is taken from Burtt's edition.
31. William Harvey, *Movement of the Heart and Blood in Animals,* translated by Kenneth J. Franklin (Oxford: Blackwell, 1957).
32. William Harvey, *The Circulation of the Blood,* translated by Kenneth J. Franklin (Oxford: Blackwell, 1958), pp. 44–45.
33. "Prius in confesso esse debet, quod sit, antequam propter quid, inquirendum." *Ibid.,* pp. 135–36. Franklin's generally superb translation does not, I feel, convey quite the precise inference I wish to draw from this passage.
34. Harvey, *Movement of the Heart,* p. 7.
35. *Circulation of the Blood,* p. 55, also pp. 144–45.
36. *Movement of the Heart,* p. 44.
37. *Ibid.,* pp. 9–21.
38. *Ibid.,* p. 167.
39. *Ibid.,* p. 61.
40. *Ibid.,* p. 51.
41. *Ibid.,* p. 80. Italics not in text.
42. *Novum Organum,* Book I, Aphorism 70 (Burtt, p. 48; *Works,* III, 353).
43. Friedrich Hoffmann, *Medicina rationalis systematica* (2d ed.; 8 vols. in 4; Halle, 1729–39).
44. *Novum Organum,* Book I, Aphorism 64 (Burtt, p. 44; *Works,* III, 351).
45. *Ibid.,* Aphorism 54 (Burtt, p. 39; *Works,* III, 349).
46. "Quemadmodum ii, qui in veritate inquirenda, omni posito prejudicio, nullius opinionis servi sunt, sed libero animo solidoque judicio cuncta perpendunt, de opinionibus prudenter dubitant, nil, nisi quod clarum, facile, simplex atque intellectui planum est, amplectuntur & optima quaeque ex omnibus seligunt, laude digni sunt: ita quoque cordati medici est, nulli sectae, vel hypothesi, in totum se mancipare,

sed potius omnia suis examinare ponderibus, & quae usui sunt ac veritati consentiunt, seligere, variis opinionibus, quae perniciosarum dissensionum in praxi & theoria genetrices sunt, rejectis & prorsus repudiatis." Hoffmann, I, 30–31.

47. *Ibid.,* I, 4.

48. *Ibid.,* I, 5.

49. *Ibid.,* I, 6.

50. "Principium plane obscurum, quod nec definiri, nec concipi potest, demonstrationibus est ineptum." *Ibid.,* I, 43.

51. ". . . pigrorum ingeniorum solatia & asyla." *Ibid., loc. cit.*

52. "Vera experientia nascitur ex compluribus observationibus, magna diligentia, attentione & cura notatis, quae integram morbi historiam, cum omnibus ad rem pertinentibus circumstantiis, complectuntur, unde medicarum observationum summa patet utilitas." *Ibid.,* I, 9.

53. *Ibid., loc. cit.*

54. *Ibid.,* p. 11.

55. *Ibid.,* p. 10.

56. *Ibid.,* pp. 11–12.

57. *Ibid.,* p. 19.

58. "Attenta observatione discimus, motum omnium mutationum in corporeis causam esse, atque motu quoque vitae ac sanitatis fundamentum contineri, ipsas morborum causas vix alio modo, quam motu, in corporis nostri solidas & fluidas partes agere, neque medicamenta aliter, quam motu, operationes exserere. Qua de causa in explanadis medicis rebus inque remediorum viribus explicandis, ad motum principaliter, deinde ad mobile, sive dispositionem corporum ipsasque vias, respiciendum esse existimamus." *Ibid.,* I, 19.

59. *Ibid.,* I, 55–56.

60. "Ergo vita & mors mechanice fiunt, & nonnisi a causis mechanicis, physicis & quae ex necessitate agunt, dependent." *Ibid.,* I, 75.

61. *Ibid.,* I, 76.

62. "Motus itaque, quo omne, quicquid fit & evenit in corpore nostro, perficitur, & quo etiam medicus in demonstrando uti debet, nullus alius est, quam contractio & expansio, sive, secundum Graecos, systole et diastole fibrarum nervearum & musculosarum & quae ex his contexti sunt, cordis atque arteriarum omniumque ductuum, cujus beneficio omnis generis fluida, per innumerabiles & varios canales, in orbem moventur . . ." *Ibid.,* I, 48.

63. Alexander Berg, "Die Lehre von der Faser als Form- und Funktionselement des Organismus," *Virchows Archiv für pathologisch Anatomie,* CCCIX (1942), 333.

64. "Neque aliud in sanandis morbis quaerere debet medicus, quam, ut causas morbificas earumque noxios effectus per congrua remedia removendo, liberum sanguinis motum atque circuitum restituat." Hoffmann, I, 49.

65. *Ibid.,* p. 73.

66. *Ibid.,* p. 68.

67. *Ibid.,* pp. 66–67.

68. *Ibid.*, p. 63.

69. *Ibid.*, pp. 57–58.

70. *Ibid.*, p. 83.

71. "Ergo non mens, non anima sensitiva, adaequata & perpetua ac proxima causa est motuum vitalium systoles & diastoles, quibus omnes actiones secundum & praeter naturam celebrantur: sed fluidum tenuissimum, calidum, elasticum, quod in minimis membranarum ac nervorum tubulis & in ipso sanguine continetur, horum motuum, adeoque vitae, sanitatis & morborum causa est." *Ibid.*, p. 85.

72. *Ibid.*, pp. 80–81.

73. "Sanguis itaque rectissime thesaurus vitae & animae vehiculum ac vinculus ejus cum corpore dicitur." *Ibid.*, p. 81. To translate "anima" in this context I chose the English term "vital principle."

74. *Ibid.*, p. 92.

75. *Ibid.*, p. 95.

76. G. H. Whipple, F. S. Robscheit, and C. W. Hooper, "Blood Regeneration Following Simple Anemia: IV. Influence of Meat, Liver and Various Extractives, Alone or Combined With Standard Diets," *American Journal of Physiology*, LIII (1920), 236; F. S. Robscheit-Robbins and G. H. Whipple, "Blood Regeneration in Severe Anemia: II. Favorable Influences of Liver, Heart and Skeletal Muscle in Diet," *ibid.*, LXXII (1925), 408.

77. Hoffmann, *op. cit.*, I, 95.

78. *Ibid.*, p. 96.

79. "Sanguis in tubulo vitreo per accuratius microscopium quando inspicitur, apparet ut aqua, cui innumeri rubicundi globuli innatant, qui nihil aliud sunt, quam gelatinosa & sulphurea sanguinis pars, quae per motum et intestinam agitationem divisa, globosam assumit figuram. Omnia enim heterogenea, in alieno fluido contenta & quassata, globosam figuram accipiunt. Et quo magis hi globuli sunt divisi, adeoque minores et copiosioras, eo sanguis fluidior, floridior & ad circulum vitalem tuendum optior existit: quo majores vero & pauciores hi globuli sunt, eo crassior ac nigricantior est." *Ibid.*, pp. 100–101.

80. *Ibid.*, pp. 88–89.

81. *Ibid.*, p. 99.

82. *Ibid.*, pp. 62–63.

83. *Ibid.*, p. 63.

84. *Ibid.*, p. 64.

CHAPTER V. CELL THEORY, KEY TO MODERN MEDICINE

1. John R. Baker, "The Cell-Theory: A Restatement, History, and Critique, Part I," *Quarterly Journal of Microscopical Science*, LXXXIX (1948), 107.

2. A. Wolf, *A History of Science, Technology, and Philosophy in the 16th and 17th Centuries* (London: Allen & Unwin, 1950), pp. 73, 416.

3. Arthur Hughes, *A History of Cytology* (London and New York: Abelard-Schumann, 1959), Plates I, VII.

4. Baker, *op. cit.;* "Part II," *ibid.,* XC (1949), 87; "Part III. The Cell as a Morphologic Unit," *ibid.,* XCIII (1952), 157; "Part IV. The Multiplication of Cells," *ibid.,* XCIV (1953), 407; "Part V. The Multiplication of Nuclei," *ibid.,* XCVI (1955), 449; Hughes, *op. cit.;* Arnold Rice Rich, "The Place of R.-J.-H. Dutrochet in the Development of Cell Theory, *"Bulletin of the Johns Hopkins Hospital,* XXXIX (1926), 330; Hans G. Schlumberger, "Origins of the Cell Concept in Pathology," *Archives of Pathology,* XXXVII (1944), 396; Marc Klein, *Histoire des origines de la théorie cellulaire* (Paris: Hermann et Cie., 1936).

5. For a general analysis of these concepts, see Lester S. King, *The Medical World of the Eighteenth Century* (Chicago: University of Chicago Press, 1958), pp. 67–70.

6. *Dr. Boerhaave's Academical Lectures on the Theory of Physic, Being a Genuine Translation of his Institutes and Explanatory Comment* (6 vols.; 2d ed.; London: W. Innys, 1751–57), II, 173–74.

7. F. J. Cole, "The History of Anatomical Injections," in *Studies in the History and Method of Science,* ed. Charles Singer (Oxford: Clarendon Press, 1921), II, 285.

8. *Academical Lectures,* II, 218–19.

9. *Ibid.,* p. 224.

10. *Ibid.,* p. 91.

11. *Ibid.,* pp. 105–10.

12. *Ibid.,* p. 121.

13. *Ibid.,* p. 97; see also pp. 90–104.

14. *Ibid.,* p. 151; see also pp. 150–60.

15. *Ibid.,* p. 157.

16. Cole, *op. cit.*

17. *Academical Lectures,* II, 215.

18. *Ibid.,* p. 238.

19. *Ibid.,* pp. 241–42.

20. *Ibid.,* p. 259.

21. Marcel Florkin, *Naissance et déviation de la théorie cellulaire dans l'oeuvre de Théodore Schwann* (Paris: Hermann, 1960).

22. Rembert Watermann, *Theodor Schwann, Leben und Werk* (Düsseldorf: L. Schwann, 1960).

23. Th. Schwann, *Microscopical Researches into the Accordance in the Structure and Growth of Animals and Plants,* translated by Henry Smith (London: Sydenham Society, 1847).

24. See note 4, above.

25. Hughes, *op. cit.,* p. 35.

26. M. J. Schleiden, *Contributions to Phytogenesis,* translated from the German, in Schwann (1847), pp. 230–63.

27. Schwann, *op. cit.,* pp. xiv, xv; Florkin, *op. cit.,* p. 62; Watermann, *op. cit.,* pp. 98–99.

28. Hughes, *op. cit.,* p. 35.

29. *Ibid.*, p. 12.
30. Schwann, *op. cit.*, p. 21.
31. *Ibid.*, pp. 36–37.
32. Schleiden, *op. cit.*, p. 233.
33. *Ibid.*, pp. 234–35.
34. Hughes, *op. cit.*, p. 39.
35. Schleiden, *op. cit.*, p. 237.
36. *Ibid.*, p. 238.
37. Schwann, *op. cit.*, p. 39.
38. *Ibid.*, p. 71.
39. Alexander Berg, "Die Lehre von der Faser als Form- und Funktionselement des Organismus," *Virchows Archiv für pathologische Anatomie,* CCCIX (1942), 333.
40. Schwann, *op. cit.*, p. 130.
41. *Ibid.*, p. 165.
42. *Ibid.*, p. 71, italics mine.
43. *Ibid.*, p. 120.
44. *Ibid.*, p. 108.
45. *Ibid.*, p. xvii.
46. *Ibid.*, p. 95.
47. *Ibid.*, p. 39.
48. R. Virchow, "Rokitansky, '*Handbuch der allgemeinen pathologischen Anatomie,*'" *Medicinische Zeitung,* 1846, pp. 237–38 and 243–44. This review is reproduced in part in W. Becker, *Rudolph Virchow, Eine biographische Studie* (Berlin: S. Karger, 1891), pp. 46–51.
49. Lester S. King, "The Medical Revolution," *Quarterly Bulletin, Northwestern University Medical School,* XXXIV (1960), 358.
50. Carl Rokitansky, *A Manual of Pathological Anatomy,* translated by W. E. Swaine, G. E. Day, C. H. Moore, E. Sieveking (4 vols.; London: The Sydenham Society, 1849–54), I, 85.
51. *Ibid.*, pp. 80, 88–89, 98–101.
52. *Ibid.*, pp. 133–40.
53. *Ibid.*, p. 143.
54. *Ibid.*, p. 144.
55. *Ibid.*, p. 145.
56. *Ibid.*, p. 134.
57. *Ibid.*, p. 377.
58. *Ibid.*, p. 293.
59. *Ibid.*, p. 300.
60. *Ibid.*, p. 304.
61. *Ibid.*, p. 91.
62. *Ibid.*, p. 362.
63. *Ibid.*, p. 370.
64. *Ibid.*, p. 363.
65. *Ibid.*, p. 370.
66. *Ibid.*, p. 372.
67. *Ibid.*, pp. 324–25.

68. Erwin H. Ackerknecht, *Rudolph Virchow, Doctor, Statesman, Anthropologist* (Madison: University of Wisconsin Press, 1953).
69. Virchow, *op. cit.* (1846), p. 237; Becker, *op. cit.*, p. 47.
70. "Standpoints in Scientific Medicine," in *Disease, Life, and Man, Selected Essays by Rudolph Virchow,* translated by Lelland J. Rather (Stanford, Cal.: Stanford University Press, 1958), pp. 33–34.
71. "Cellular Pathology," *ibid.*, p. 72.
72. Baker, *op. cit.* ("Part IV").
73. *Ibid.*, p. 435.
74. Walter Pagel, *Virchow und die Grundlagen der Medizin des XIX Jahrhunderts* (Jena: Gustav Fischer, 1931); "The Speculative Basis of Modern Pathology. Jahn, Virchow, and the Philosophy of Pathology," *Bulletin of the History of Medicine,* XVIII (1945), 1.
75. Virchow, *Cellular Pathology, as Based upon Physiological and Pathological Histology,* translated from the second edition by Frank Chance (New York: DeWitt, n.d. [1860]).
76. Ackerknecht, *op. cit.*, p. 33.
77. Virchow, "Ueber die Reform der pathologischen und therapeutischen Anschauungen durch die Mikroskopischen Untersuchungen," *Archiv für pathologische Anatomie,* I (1847), 217–18; in this connection see Ackerknecht, *op. cit.*, p. 58.
78. *Cellular Pathology,* pp. 57, 69, 77.
79. *Ibid.*, p. 42.
80. "Man kann daher mit geringen Einschränkungen in der That *an die Stelle des früheren Blastems und späteren Exsudats, der ursprünglich plastischen Lymphe der Alten, das Bindegewebe mit seinem Aequivalenten als den gemeinschaftlichen Keimstock des Körpers setzen,* und von ihm aus die eigentliche Entwickelung der späteren Theile ableiten." Virchow, *Die Cellularpathologie in ihrer Begründung auf physiologische und pathologische Gewebelehre.* (Berlin: Hirschwald, 1858), p. 355. In the English translation by Frank Chance, *op. cit.*, p. 441, this passage is rendered in what seems to me a very barbarous fashion, and I offer my own translation.
81. *Cellular Pathology,* pp. 182–83.
82. *Ibid.*, p. 188, italics mine.
83. *Ibid.*, p. 83.
84. *Ibid.*, pp. 494–95.
85. *Ibid.*, p. 490.
86. *Ibid.*, p. 489.
87. *Ibid.*, p. 497.
88. *Ibid.*, p. 466.
89. *Ibid.*, p. 453.
90. *Ibid.*, p. 489.
91. *Ibid.*, p. 465.
92. *Ibid.*, p. 499.
93. Virchow, *Die Krankhaften Geschwulste* (3 vols.; Berlin: Hirschwald, 1863–65).

94. *Cellular Pathology*, p. 111.
95. *Ibid.*, p. 115.
96. *Ibid.*, p. 117.
97. *Ibid.*, pp. 117–18.
98. *Ibid.*, p. 124.
99. *Ibid.*, p. 134.
100. *Ibid.*, p. 114.

EPILOGUE

1. William Osler, "Medicine in the Nineteenth Century," in *Aequanimitas* (3d ed.; Philadelphia: P. Blakiston's Son & Co., 1932), p. 219.
2. Lester S. King, "Dr. Koch's Postulates," *Journal of the History of Medicine and Allied Sciences*, VII (1952), 350.
3. Osler, "Internal Medicine as a Vocation," *op. cit.*, p. 137.
4. Linus Pauling, Harvey A. Itano, S. J. Singer, and Ibert C. Wells, "Sickle Cell Anemia, a Molecular Disease," *Science*, CX (1949), 543.
5. *Ibid.*, p. 547.
6. G. W. Beadle, "Biochemical Genetics," *Chemical Reviews*, XXXVII (1945), 15.
7. *Ibid.*, p. 61.
8. V. M. Ingram, "A Specific Chemical Difference Between the Globins of Normal Human and Sickle-cell Anaemia Hemoglobin," *Nature*, CLXXVIII (1956), 793.
9. Herbert Lehmann and J. A. M. Agar, "The Hemoglobinopathies and Thalassemia," in *The Metabolic Basis of Inherited Disease*, ed. John B. Stansbury, James B. Wyngaarden, and Donald S. Frederickson (New York, Toronto, London: McGraw-Hill, 1960), pp. 1095–97.
10. David Yi-Yung Hsia, *Inborn Errors of Metabolism* (Chicago: Year Book Publishers, 1959); Stansbury *et al.*, *op. cit.*
11. John M. Allen (ed.), *The Molecular Control of Cellular Activity* (New York: McGraw-Hill Book Company, 1962).

Index

251